TO BE A SURGEON

TO BE A SURGEON

Richard Furman, M.D., F.A.C.S.

FREDERICK FELL PUBLISHERS, INC.
New York, New York

Altered names conceal the identities of persons mentioned in this book.

Copyright © 1982 by Richard Furman, M.D.

For information address:

FREDERICK FELL PUBLISHERS, INC.
386 Park Avenue South
New York, New York 10016

Library of Congress Catalog Card Number: 81-68914
International Standard Book Number: 0-8119-0444-X

MANUFACTURED IN THE UNITED STATES OF AMERICA

1 2 3 4 5 6 7 8 9 0

Published simultaneously in Canada by Fitzhenry & Whiteside Limited, Toronto

Dedicated to my parents,
who have given me more than money can buy:
direction when needed, advice when wanted,
and love in their hearts forever.

FOREWORD

No matter what our position in life, we need to set goals and learn how to achieve those goals. For Dr. Richard Furman, it took many years of hard, dedicated work to complete medical school and surgical training. To achieve the position of surgeon, he set goals for himself that he could neither alter nor deviate from if he was to be successful—and he established a goal structure that proved itself. This structure not only is beneficial to a surgeon, but also is workable, I have found, in any field of endeavor.

I was challenged not long ago by Dr. Furman and his brother, Lowell, to help organize a group that would send volunteer physicians, four to six weeks at a time, to mission hospitals in the Third World countries. Immediately, questions arose in my mind. How does one set up such an organization? How does one sell such an idea to a physician: leave home and practice, and embark (at his or her own expense) thousands of miles to a Third World country to serve as a relief physician in a mission hospital?

My college education was concentrated in business—I had taken courses in sales, management, accounting, and statistics. There was nothing in my formal education, therefore, that taught me how to establish such an organization. But I did know how to ask questions and seek answers. Setting our goal structures early and starting with a list of sixteen physicians, we placed our goals under God's guidance. Today, two years later, we are achieving tremendous success—over one thousand physicians interested in the program, with 160 directly participating.

We could not have reached these figures without setting goals and working to achieve those goals. Goal-setting gives you a purpose, and a yardstick, so to speak, to measure your performance. Without it you flounder, waste money, and expend too much valuable, irreplaceable energy. Our new goals include doubling our volunteer physician-participation in two years!

TO BE A SURGEON has been a source of personal encouragement, a book that has pointed out areas of my life in which I am weak and need to be strengthened with a clear goal structure. Its underlying message can also stimulate *you* to reach the full potential of your life.

As you read these pages, my prayer is that you will be motivated to channel your life to a goal-setting structure, that you will set very high goals for yourself without fear of failure, and that you will be dedicated to the point that enables you to obtain all out of life that God intended for you—and not be shortchanged in any area.

While writing this book, Dr. Furman had something extraordinary happen to him that I also experienced about the same time. This experience, about which you will read, gave a whole new perspective on goals and offered both of us new goals to work on for the rest of our lives—goals we will never tire of striving for, goals that give a purpose and meaning to life, goals that make each day worth waking up and living for. You will become a different person if you read these pages and follow the structure set before you.

I hope you enjoy this book as much as I have, and that it will encourage you to explore the horizons of a goal-setting structure.

Franklin Graham, President
Samaritan's Purse/World Medical Mission

TO BE A SURGEON

Part I

MEDICAL SCHOOL

EIGHT YEARS AGO Mrs. Avery's husband died of a heart attack, and since that time she has surrounded herself with medical students. We are not physicians but she feels safer, I guess. There are three large rooms upstairs. The rent is cheap, the accommodations clean and, best of all, we are left alone and it is quiet. I choose the corner room with its big bed, big desk, and two windows where studying looks natural. My desk would be worth seven hundred at an antique shop, yet it is only a piece of unmatched furniture left over from some partially successful insurance business of Mrs. Avery's husband's. I can tell the felt pad on the top of the desk is at least three years old from the reminders and dates scribbled in the corners. I lean back in the old hardwood chair and stare at nothing in particular on the desk in front of me.

My eyes stop at something underlined in the upper right hand corner of the felt pad: SET YOUR GOALS HIGH. I suppose every college student who has ever been accepted to medical school worked on the goal of being accepted.

I remember back to my senior year in high school when I made the decision to go to medical school. That was a major decision in my life, and a major goal. Once that goal was decided on, I never thought of changing it. No matter how bad the odds became, I never ever played with the idea of changing that goal. I believe that is the basis of being here today: a major decision, a major goal.

I reach for my pen and scribble on the few blank spaces on the felt pad under SET YOUR GOALS HIGH: MAJOR GOAL: Set it and Never Change It.

I remember my high school teacher sincerely advising me against a pre-medical curriculum in college because I was barely passing chemistry and we both knew chemistry would be a major concentration of pre-medical studies at college. To me, this only brought about the realization that in order to reach my goal of being accepted to medical school, I had to excel in chemistry once in college. The

— 3 —

day prior to starting college I sat in my room at a desk as I do today and set another goal: To excel in chemistry. This would be necessary in order to reach my major goal of being accepted to medical school. This goal of excelling in chemistry was directly related to the major goal but was *intermediate* in the span of time of college. I realized at that time that if I did not obtain this *intermediate* goal, the *major* goal would never be reached.

I lean forward and write again on the felt pad just under MAJOR GOAL: Set It and Never Change It: INTERMEDIATE GOAL: Necessary to Reach Major Goal.

I begin to see a definite structure to the goals set in reaching medical school. First came the major goal of being accepted to medical school. Then came the intermediate goal of excelling in that first chemistry course in order to reach the major goal. The intermediate goal did not seem nearly so prestigious nor glamorous as the major goal, but somehow I understood the importance of that goal even though in reality the intermediate goal was more important than the major goal because it was closer to the present time, closer to something I would have to do very soon. However, it was not until the second night at college, having attended the first chemistry class, that I happened on the cornerstone of the goal structure I would follow in the remaining college courses. It was the second night I realized that making an excellent grade in chemistry depended on what I did that night. I had the feeling of impending doom or impending excellence. The outcome of the entire goal structure depended on the action I took *immediately*. And that action meant that I had to sit down and study *now* and not go with friends or take a break or practice for the intramural football team. My major goal, my intermediate goal and, in essence, my goal structure depended on what I did, not tomorrow, not in the morning, not later tonight, but immediately.

I lean forward and add to the goal structure that has proven successful in getting me into medical school:

MAJOR GOAL: Set It and Never Change It
INTERMEDIATE GOAL: Necessary to Reach Major Goal
IMMEDIATE GOAL: Right Now, Get It Done

This was an excellent structure to get me to medical school, a secret that was hard bought. I decide to follow this same structure through medical training. I pick up a small, black, pocketsized notebook and write a new set of goals for a new chapter in my life for easy daily reference. On the first page I write, MAJOR GOAL: Become a surgeon. On the second page, INTERMEDIATE GOAL: Successfully complete anatomy and histology. These are my first two courses and will let me and everyone else know whether I am capable of completing medical school. On the third page I write, IMMEDIATE GOAL: Set study time for each day and never depart from it.

I decide to carry this notebook with me in my lab coat pocket tomorrow morning and write down any new immediate goals that I may realize as necessary for succeeding in my intermediate goal of getting through anatomy and histology successfully. I will call the notebook my *Goal's Rule Book.*

I begin the first day of medical school with all the apprehensions and uncertainty a person can endure, my entire future at stake. My schedule shows four months of anatomy in the mornings and histology in the afternoons. In keeping with the immediate goal, I write in my *Goal's Rule Book*: "I resolve to spend every minute of my life for the next thirty days either studying, eating, or sleeping. Nothing else. I will make no telephone calls, write no letters, attend no movies; think of nothing but anatomy and histology for this period of time." The first test in anatomy will be in one month.

Between anatomy and histology, anatomy is the more difficult course, claiming ten times more victims—those who wash out the first three months of school—and requiring three times the amount of study.

The first morning of classes arrives, and I meekly enter a huge lab that contains the cadavers, bodies that have been preserved solely for dissection by medical students. Entering the room I feel confident, but yet there is that small twinge of insecurity concerning whether I can learn all there is to know about the anatomy of the human body.

The freshman class numbers one hundred. I try to size up as many of my fellow students as I can as we crowd into the anatomy lab. A few are laughing and joking, but for the most part everyone appears about as uneasy as I feel. We are motioned to the front of the room where Dr. Glenn, the head of the department, is arranging papers on a clip board and getting ready to speak. I doubt I will ever forget this moment. The odor of the cadavers is indescribable, plastic sheets cover the bodies, plastic aprons, one for each student, lie over the bodies, and two jars of petroleum jelly are set on the portion of the cadaver I guess to be the abdomen. There is an excitement in the room that has no comparison.

Dr. Glenn speaks: "This morning you will be split into groups of four and draw lots for the bodies." He paces up and down in his long white coat which looks as if he had slept in it for a week. Even sitting three rows back, I can detect that it has the same odor of the cadavers, an almost putrid smell. As a matter of fact, everything in the room smells like the cadavers; the floor, the old wooden tables the bodies lie on, the high stools around the tables, and the bookstands which hold the atlases with pictures of different parts of the body to be dissected. But, after ten minutes the odor becomes less noticeable; all attention is focused on Dr. Glenn. "The small skinny ones are the best to get. Some have arms missing, some have been operated on, some are fat; but you are stuck with the number you draw. If anyone doesn't like his cadaver, I will bring up 'the China-man.' He weights 305 pounds and is five feet two inches tall. We have preserved him for eight years now and won't hesitate to use him if someone complains about the condition of his cadaver." This statement puts us all at the mercy of fate. Whatever number we draw, we have to keep.

The dissecting group I elect to be with consists of three of my friends. We attended the same college and were classmates in most of our pre-med courses with the exception of Bill Warren who was three years ahead of the rest of us. Persistence made it possible for him to be here. We are all rooming together, and each of us has agreed to do nothing but study for the first month. We would give any earthly belongings in return for a good cadaver, but that will be determined by lot. We elect Bill to draw for the cadaver. We get table number six. Anxiously, we walk over and pull back the sheet.

"Not a bit over eighty-five pounds," Bill boasts. Sure enough, there is the cadaver we will be living with for the next four months, a Negro female, about eighty years old with almost no fat on her body to speak of. We stand motionless and stare at her without speaking. Her skin is dry and feels unnatural. We are instructed to rub two jars of petroleum jelly on her from her toes to the holes in her ears to keep the skin from cracking. Her hair and fingernails look perfectly natural, but her eyes are dull, the whites cloudy. Her tongue lies unnaturally—slightly stiff and very dry. She has pierced ears and skinny fingers with wrinkled skin. We couldn't have picked a better cadaver if given the choice of the entire room. We slap Bill on the back and congratulate him as if he had just won a million dollar sweepstakes. It brings a good feeling knowing there will be less time spent on dissecting, with more time left for review at the end of the day.

"She looks like her name ought to be 'Minnie,'" Pokie says. Pokie is the nickname we have given Larry Pike because everything he does is slow and deliberate. He walks slowly, eats slowly, talks slowly; everything he does is slow except his thinking. He is a rapid learner and quick to grasp new ideas. He has the highest scholastic average of anyone in our group and will have no difficulty getting through medical school. Even though we kid him about his slow ways, we all have some envy of his quick learning ability. Minnie is her new name and Minnie is what we begin to call her.

The days pass quickly as we enter the routine of freshman medical students. I realize something new to write in the back of my goals book that I am carrying around. It is a realization that becoming a surgeon is something I think of when I first awaken and the last thing when I go to sleep. I think that may be one essential factor in making a dream come true. I write: A major goal is something you first awaken to and the last thing you think of as you go to sleep.

During the first few days, everyone remains tense as each of us actually puts a knife to "Minnie's" skin and cuts through the tissues. Before long, we become more relaxed and as our confidence builds, our seriousness slackens.

This is the time I feel the need to push. The "new" has worn off. Some of the students are beginning to talk about a program they saw on television the night before, an occasional one talks of a movie he went to, another spent two hours after dinner shooting pool at the fraternity house. There is definitely a relaxed attitude creeping into the class and I must guard against becoming a part of it. I need to keep a clear view of my goals in preparing for the first test to the very best of my ability.

I also remind myself of Bill Warren. The odds of being accepted to medical school are about twenty to one. Only about five percent of those who apply actually are accepted. Bill beat the percentages by persistence. He was rejected three years in a row before being accepted. What he lacked in grades, he made up in persistence. That has to be one of the secrets of obtaining goals. Bill's goal was not reached initially but he never changed his mind. He was going to enter medical school if it took twenty years. He didn't say he would make it to medical school if there wasn't a death in the family. He didn't say he would make it to medical school if he didn't wreck his car. He didn't say he would make it to medical school if he didn't run out of money. If he had not had persistence he would not have been accepted because each of those things did happen to him, he *persisted* and his goal was reached.

I again turn in the small notebook to the page labeled "Thoughts" and write PERSISTENCE: Vital to Reaching the Goal.

Closing the notebook, I realize I am somewhat more relaxed about studying and the everyday chores of school. I've even noticed I have a different attitude toward the cadaver. She is no longer a smelly old body but has taken on some character. We now greet her with "Good morning, Minnie," and always leave with "Good night, Minnie." We realize she is only a body without a spirit or soul, but after a while it seems almost as if she does sense what we are doing. Soon, it is normal to converse with "Minnie" without feeling foolish about the one-sided conversation.

"Minnie, don't you have a radial nerve?"

"I believe you are hiding your stellate ganglion and if you don't show it to me, I'll pinch your carotid artery."

I talk, Pokie talks. In due time we find her mouth will stay in the position in which we place it. If one of us feels particularly happy, we turn the corners of her mouth up and work all day on a smiling little old lady. If someone feels grouchy, down go the corners and we work in a "grouch" atmosphere.

The first four weeks pass more rapidly than any time in my life. We cover her shoulder, neck, and arm, dissect each muscle, vessel, and nerve, and no sooner do I finish studying the hand than the time arrives for our first test. I feel stunned that the showdown is actually upon me. This is the test that we hear so much about from the sophomore students. They keep shaking their heads and laughing every time one of us mentions the upcoming test, telling us studying is useless. I have noticed a slight amount of diarrhea the past three days, a sure sign my nervous system is overworking.

In only one month I have acquired full appreciation of the often quoted statement: "Getting into medical school is one thing, but staying there is something else." The pace is fast; we cover as much material in one week of medical school as we would be expected to learn in a whole quarter in college. There is no time to go over the subject four or five times in preparing for a test; the material has to be learned the first time around since there is too much covered to try to rely on recall from a cram study period the day before the exam. This first test is to cover the neck, shoulder, and arm region in minute detail. Every day, I have gone over the gross specimens assigned for the time allotted and each night reviewed the atlas and textbook covering the area I dissected that day. Our class has even paid the janitor to come back and unlock the lab on Saturdays so we could have more time to dissect the cadavers.

Now the cards are on the table. Approximately fifteen percent of the class will flunk this first anatomy test. This test is *the* deciding factor, the one material object which puts all the talk, all the speculation, all the self-esteem on the line. At last someone is going to give me a number which I can interpret any way my conscious mind will let me. If I make a low grade, my mind will tell me I will do better next time. If I make class average, my mind can tell me I am going to make it in medical school. If I make a high grade, I must strive just as hard on the next test to keep myself there.

Nine o'clock. I glance at my watch while sitting at my desk the evening prior to the test. I am not really learning anything, only staring at notes I have reviewed numerous times before. It seems almost illegally wrong to go to bed early the night before a test, but I decide sleep will be more beneficial than staring, so I go to bed and get ten hours of restful sleep.

I walk into class at eight-fifty and take a seat near the back. The cumulative result of my immediate action goals is at hand.

Numerous Right Now, Get It Done events have occurred. After supper, when to start studying?—Right Now, Get It Done; finish dissecting a particular nerve, or wait until morning when I am fresh?—Right Now, Get It Done; look up a word in the medical dictionary, or let it go?—Right Now, Get It Done; find the location of the artery in the atlas tonight, or wait and look for it tomorrow in Minnie?—Right Now, Get It Done!

The immediate goals are complete. Now lets see if the goal structure works, if it holds water, if it has laid the proper ground-work for the intermediate goal of completing anatomy and histology.

Most of the class is already present, but no one is talking. I can sense it in the air; there is some doubt in everyone's mind, not a single student here who doesn't have at least a small unsureness about this exam. But I know I am as well prepared as I will ever be. If I can't pass it, I don't need to be here. What a horrible thought— "don't need to be here." Would my mind let me set an unreachable goal? Surely I can think of some goals I would not be able to attain, no matter how hard I strived. Could it be possible? Could I have set an unreachable goal before I took that first chemistry course in college? I have to think I am going to pass this exam, finish medical school and become a surgeon, have to believe that my mind would never let me set an impossible goal. There has to be some unknown mechanism which prevents the mind from allowing one to write down an impossible goal.

I mentally write a note for my goal book. "Is it possible for a person to set an impossible goal? I think not, but I am about to find out what goals, and desire and persistence are all about. I will know a lot more about all of these about four hours from now with the test completed."

The first two hours of the test is written, covering the origin, insertion, and innervation of all the muscles in the region we have dissected. There are several discussion questions concerning the plexus of nerves in the neck and shoulder as well as what type of injury would result if a particular nerve were injured. There are other questions. Some I know completely and remember even more than is asked; some I only vaguely remember reading about.

After forty-five minutes, minutes that seem like hours, I sense movement in the room. I look up to see someone turning in his paper and leaving. I can't believe he has completed the test when I am not halfway through. I finish the test in an hour and a half, but am not about to hand it in until the two-hour limit is announced. I still have time to go over the questions once more, make sure I have not misread a question or given a wrong answer when I know the correct one. The announcement is made that time is up; everything is answered the way I intend it.

The next two hours are not only a test of intellect but also of nerves. There are twenty-five bodies, each with yellow tags attached to particular parts that have been dissected. Some are obvious, some vaguely obscure. Everyone picks a station to begin the test. The instructor stands at the head of the room with a large clock that will sound off with a loud buzz every two minutes. Each time it sounds, we move to the next station whether we have identified the tagged portion of the cadaver or not.

Look at the specimen.
Think!
Eyes closed. Try to remember!
Buzzer
Move to the next specimen.
Easy one—write it down and think back to the last one.
Think! Name of the branch of that nerve. I can't think.
Buzzer
Move to the next specimen.
Think! Think! Think! Got to come up with this one! I know this one if I can slow down and think.
Quit listening for the buzzer.
Think! Ansa hypoglossal! That's it. Write it down.
Think back to the one I missed.
I don't know it! I don't remember—No, I don't know.
Buzzer.

I near the cadaver I began with, signifying the end of the road and realize there are six blanks on my paper. I had planned to answer these as I had time to think, but that time never came. I decide to fill them in as best I remember from the little notes I have written in the margins of the answer sheet. The final buzzer sounds. The test is over.

I turn in my paper and find myself with absolutely nothing to do. I have studied so much in the past month, I couldn't possibly read anything else about medicine.

Today is Saturday, and we wouldn't start another section on our cadavers until Monday. This is the first free time I have had since beginning anatomy, and it is too nice a day not to drive 120 miles to surprise that girl I told not to expect to see me until Thanksgiving.

I notice a strange phenomena. Twenty-four hours into the weekend and I am just beginning to relax. My mind has been running in high gear for a month and it won't let me ease back into the free and easy style I was used to in college. Does this mean I will soon be geared to run at a higher speed for the rest of my life, or will I be able to slip back into a frame of mind which will allow me to waste a little time, here and there?

I quit thinking about it and begin to enjoy what little free time I do have. Harriet is so excited to see me this weekend. We have dated for a year and a half; I think it's time to get married. She is starting her junior year at college and I know we can't wait until she graduates before we get married. I haven't asked her to marry me, but I know she is thinking along the same line as I am. I decided she was the girl I would marry after our second date in college and have just assumed that it will eventually happen. Five feet, two inches and ninety-two pounds—just right. I guess the first step is to figure out how to get her education taken care of. The real problem is the fact that there is no college near the medical school. We will have to talk this situation over and come up with a workable solution before discussing it with her parents. Which is more important, our happiness or her college education?

I present the idea to Harriet. It is fun to actually start thinking along the line of marriage. We arrive at no solution to our problem, however. Sunday afternoon approaches, and it is time to quit thinking about Harriet and begin thinking about what grade I made on the anatomy test.

Monday morning comes quickly, I can feel butterflies creeping into my stomach as I walk up the steps to the anatomy class. Test papers are to be returned this afternoon. Where is my faith in my analogy of goals? As the day progresses, the butterflies worsen. I keep convincing myself, but do not feel like eating lunch. The grade curve is announced: 48–98. The papers are returned at five P.M. Big red numbers: a 9 and a 4. All I can do is stare at them. My eyes fix on the grade at the top of page one—94. Within the upper one-fourth of the class at least. The feeling is the same as when I learned I was accepted at medical school. I know now I am going to make it. This strengthens the idea that whatever I strive for I can reach. Still, I am not one hundred percent certain if this is true. I have so much ahead of me to tackle. New immediate goal: Next section of anatomy and histology, continue same study habits. Right now, get it done. I neatly write this on the "Immediate Goals" page of my book.

Immediate goals are always changing. I'll be glad when anatomy and histology are over and I can change my intermediate goal for the first time. I review the *Goal's Rule Book* again:

MAJOR GOAL: Become a surgeon.

INTERMEDIATE GOAL: Successfully complete anatomy and histology.

IMMEDIATE GOAL: Next section of anatomy and histology, continue same study habits, right now, get it done.

As time progresses, my rotation on anatomy becomes more enjoyable, less demanding. I develop a routine consisting of going to class all day, studying until twelve-thirty, going to bed, getting up and back to class. No movies, no television, no breaks—just sticking to the routine. However, a big change in original plans has developed. Each weekend I pack my books into the car and take off to see Harriet. I guess I can now call her my fiancée even though I haven't really asked her to marry me. This particular weekend is special, at least to my way of thinking. We dissected on the heart during the week, and I slip it out of the building as I leave, rationalizing the act by telling myself I want to study the valves and arteries in the heart over the weekend. But, I know the real reason is to show Harriet what a real human heart looks like inside and out. I can hardly wait to get to her house with my "surprise package" floating inside a jar of formalin.

After two and a half hours of traveling, I arrive. After the usual ritual of giving her a hug and kiss, I remove the jar from the sack to demonstrate my newly-learned knowledge of the heart.

Harriet shifts away from me and takes three steps backward.

"It's only Minnie's heart. Look, this is where the blood comes in," I authoritatively point out. "It goes from here to the lungs and back into the heart."

She shows slight interest, but it is evident I will not be able to take it out of the jar to show any of the details. I find it difficult to believe she doesn't have the interest I think she ought to. If she is to be a doctor's wife, she ought to *want* to hold a real heart; at least that's the way I look at it. However, I accept reality and place the jar back on the front seat.

As we finish dinner, Harriet and I go over the game plan we have decided to present to her folks. We decide that there is no real reason for her to finish college. What is important in our lives is our happiness, our being together. The best way to accomplish this is for Harriet to quit college, take a secretarial course, and in less than two months be typing away in someone's office. She can make enough for us to live on and after four years I'll be starting internship and making some additional money.

We get our story straight and ask her parents to sit down. I begin, "We would like to go over something with you to see what you think. We have decided that there is no real reason for Harriet to finish college. What is important in our lives is our happiness and our just being together. The best way to accomplish this is for Harriet to quit college and take a secretarial course." I pause because I can tell her father wants to say something.

"I have always wanted Harriet to finish college. I think she should."

For some reason, the rest of my story doesn't want to come out of my mouth. He hasn't said we can't get married; he won't say that. But, he has told us exactly what he is thinking. We end the discussion fairly coldly with no one knowing how not to say anything wrong. Harriet and I will have to reconsider our plans. So I return to class and we postpone any decisions for the time being.

I finish anatomy and histology as the newness of being in medical school wears off. With most of the excitement and enthusiasm vanishing, it's beginning to be more like an over demanding post-graduate school. I find some of the courses only vaguely related to what I think necessary to become a doctor, much less a surgeon. I force myself to study by remembering the entire gamut must be taken, and passed, in order to receive a degree. On this, I have to rationalize. Many of the courses do not pertain in the slightest to surgery. I am not particularly interested in some of them, will never use the knowledge once the final exam is over. Why not relax and just get by, rather than knock myself out for grades? I must reassess my major goal, intermediate goal, and immediate goal before I can decide what action to take. Major—surgery, Intermediate—whatever course I am taking, Immediate—knowledge of a course I'm not interested in.

What do I do with courses that are not of interest to me? Can I utilize my *Goal's Rule Book* to help answer this question? Perhaps I will have to come up with a new rule to insert into the book that will deal with this situation. I am sure it will become a greater problem as school progresses.

To analyze the problem below skin depth, I consider the known goals. MAJOR: To become a surgeon. Now, to accomplish this I must be accepted to a superb residency training program. To accomplish that, I must be accepted to a superb internship. Now to the truth of the matter. Internship acceptance depends on two items: recommendations and grades.

Good grades are easier to obtain if I have a genuine interest in the course. Therefore, I need to somehow develop an interest in a course I am completely disinterested in.

How?

AGGRESSIVE POSITIVE THINKING. This will be the only way. Any negative thoughts about a course will ruin it for me. I must erase the negatives as they appear and replace them with positives. I have to seek the good points in the professor, the book, the hours spent in class, and so forth. This will become my secret to control my mind in order to obtain good grades in uninteresting courses. Attack them with positiveness of mind and beat them with repeated attacks. Just like the proverbial bad apple in a barrel, the negative thought out, and replaced with a positive thought. I jot on the "thoughts" page in my book: POSITIVENESS OF MIND: Beat the negatives. Replace negatives with positives.

I move on to the studies of pathology, physiology, some pharmacology, as well as a few minor courses to fill any time slots left vacant. The first year goes well, and I start on the second year. I find I have much less enthusiasm now than I had the first day of medical school. I have to rely on the goal system of study more and more. But it is working. I cannot live on enthusiasm alone.

Harriet and I discuss our marriage situation. This first year has passed so quickly. She is now only one year away from graduation. We decide that she should finish. We are somewhat reluctant but know that there is some virtue in her completing what is begun. We decide to write each other every day. As I drive back to medical school, this weekend comes to a close. However, one thought is certain in my mind; we will be married. As far as setting a date, I am also certain when the marriage will take place. That is simple—look up the date of Harriet's graduation, and we will be married the following weekend. I reach Mrs. Avery's upstairs apartment, take a seat at the desk and start preparing for new classes in the morning.

I begin studies in parasitology, biochemistry, hematology, introduction to clinical medicine, and several courses to bridge the gap between basic sciences and actually treating the patient. The first part of this year turns out to be a gradual transition from all book work to a minute amount of time being spent actually seeing patients. It seems too gradual to me. It is six months into the year, and I am anxious to end looking at books and start looking at patients. I haven't even seen a patient, much less talked to or touched one. All I do is read until it's coming out of my ears, then go to class, take notes, study the thick medical books on my desk. I am introduced to people as being a medical student, which immediately sets off a chain reaction of some ailment either they themselves have, or some friend or relative has. I do not know any more about the ailments and diseases of the body than a biology major in college. Yet, I have finished one-and-a-half years of medical school and am expected to have the knowledge of a practicing physician. I want to start learning something about patients, about sick people, about the treatment of at least the more common diseases. I am tired of just reading how the body works, how it is put together, medications that can be used. I am ready to start applying my knowledge, all of the learning compartments of my brain are overflowing . . . saturated . . . supersaturated. I try to make myself realize it's all part of the system.

Lamar Owens is not as concerned with such thoughts as I. He has much more to think about; being on the fence, of passing or failing. I attended college with Lamar who had excellent grades, but who for some reason began having real difficulty scholastically soon after starting medical school. It has been a tough, almost terrifying, experience for him. This is verified by the fact he vomits every morning as soon as he is awake enough to realize he is in medical school and has to go to classes. What makes someone go through such torment? He is not enjoying even sixty seconds a day of his life. Why does he continue this way? He has a terrible life. I confront him with the question. Desire. The only thing that keeps Lamar getting up every morning and going to class is desire. He says so himself. I think about that.

DESIRE.

It is not the type of desire you hear one speak of when a college student says: "I would give anything to be a doctor." And all the while he is having a good time and making C's. He desires to become a doctor, but he does not desire it the way Lamar does.

As I think through the subject, I begin to realize that this special desire is what it takes to accomplish day to day immediate actions. We all have a goal, but the difference lies in who does something about it. Lamar's compelling desire is the difference between what he dreams of becoming and what he actually becomes.

This new finding impresses me enough to jot it down in my goal's book. COMPELLING DESIRE: the Necessary Force between Wanting and Having.

The year ends, both Lamar and I pass, but each with a different psychological reaction to our grades. He paid the price of compelling desire and will be rewarded for it. I am sure he will find a spot in medicine that he likes.

Medical school is basically divided into two segments. The first two years consisting mostly of study from book and classwork, and the last two years devoted to the clinical aspect of becoming a doctor, spent working with patients. I look back on the subclinical years as one hundred percent work. I learned much but am eager to get into the hospital, work the wards, get in the operating room, learn from residents. Now the time has come to take a big step in becoming a doctor; I move into the hospital. My major goal remains the same— Become a surgeon. My intermediate goal centers on completing medical school. Now is the time to change my immediate actions from thinking primarily of books to that of adding patients to the books.

June 6, the dream becomes reality. Harriet and I become man and wife. The long awaited honeymoon ends all too quickly, and the time has come to begin the exciting clinical years of school. We find a small garage apartment. Our bedroom is hardly big enough to call a room. Our double bed is pushed against one wall, and you have to turn sideways to walk between the other side of the bed and the wall.

"Why did you choose this small room to be our bedroom?" Harriet asks as we move our furniture in. "The other room would let us walk on both sides of the bed and would make it much easier to make up the bed."

"The tin roof," I reply. "There is a tin-roofed shed just outside the window in the small room. You can't beat the sound of rain beating on a tin roof for a good night's sleep. I even stuck a piece of tin in my window when I was in college so I could hear the rain. You'll see, you will like it."

"O.K., if it means that much to you, I guess I can make the bed up with it against the wall."

We finally get what little bit of furniture we have moved in and settle down for our first night in our new home. We talk of the coming year.

"You know that once classes begin we won't be able to spend much time together. I'll be on call at the hospital every third night and will need to study the other two."

Harriet smiles and replies, "Just being here is going to be so much better than last year. At least we'll have your study breaks and weekends to call our own."

It is certainly a nicer life with Harriet as my wife, and such a sweet girl to come home to. It is going to be an exciting year.

This year will consist of rotations devoted to certain specialities. One of these, internal medicine, seems to be the epitome of medical science; detailed work-ups of patients with all the special studies that are at the finger tips of the internist. New medicines are being used daily. The field seems wide open for anyone who is willing to give three extra years after internship to study the more unusual types of diseases.

Obstetrics and gynecology is another field I will rotate through this year. Some surgery is performed, but is limited to that of the female organs. I would rather be able to operate on all the organs in the abdomen if I am to operate at all.

I will also rotate through pediatrics, but doubt my disposition will allow me to be a pediatrician.

Obstetrics and gynecology is my first clinical rotation. At least, I am on my way to becoming a "real" doctor. I am assigned to the city-county hospital for the first part of the rotation. There are numerous charity cases, and most of these deliveries are done by the interns. It doesn't take long to find that the student is low man on the totem pole, even lower than the nurses since most of the nurses have been working on O.B. for years and delivering babies is second nature to them. Much of the practical work of delivering babies will be learned from them.

Our group completes the usual first day orientation, and is about to go eat dinner when we are told to report to the delivery room immediately for our assignments and introduction. Just as we enter, a woman lets out a yell so loud that we stop in our tracks, looking at one another as if someone ought to do something. We are told she is only having labor pain which will soon end. The intern introduces himself and instructs me and three fellow students to get into scrub suits in preparation for assisting with deliveries. We are designated to be "on call" tonight. The rest are free to leave, but everyone is so anxious to see a delivery, the entire group of sixteen changes into scrub suits and stays. Soon, a patient is wheeled into the delivery room as we curiously gather around. I am actually going to see a real live patient deliver a real live baby! This is real genuine medicine; nothing artificial, nothing to read about, just "doing." The intern scrubs his hands hastily, quickly puts on a sterile gown while the nurses place the woman on the delivery table. One nurse puts restraints on the patient's wrists, another places her feet and legs in stirrups. The contractions are coming at short intervals and with each, the patient writhes around on the table and moans continuously.

"Go ahead and give her the Demerol," says the intern as he makes his way to the foot of the delivery table. The nurse injects the pain medication. She has already prepped the vaginal region with surgical soap and has placed drapes around the site of the delivery. To one side of the intern is a stand about the size of a kitchen table which is covered with a sterile sheet. On it is an array of instruments, sutures, needles, basins, suction bulb, test tubes, sponges, umbilical cord clamps, and forceps. The Demoral has been given, but it seems not to have had any effect by all the noise the patient is making. The intern picks up a needle and syringe, fills it with Xylocaine and proceeds to inject the numbing medication into the top portion of the birth canal. The contractions are coming just a few seconds apart, and suddenly I see black hair on the baby's head making its appearance. For five minutes the patient continues to contract, but it doesn't seem as though the delivery is making any progress. The intern becomes nervous and mutters, "She's having her first delivery, and the head is rotated; going to have to turn the baby."

I don't know if this is serious or not, but I become more concerned as I watch perspiration begin to appear on the intern's forehead as he begins to move a little quicker and more abruptly than he has been. All attention focuses on him, and somehow the noise and fuss coming from the mother recedes in my mind, even though only a few minutes ago all I could think of was how much suffering and pain she was having and could not see how in the world any doctor could concentrate on delivering a baby with all that going on. Now, the intern takes center stage. I concentrate on his performance only.

He persists at turning the baby in the womb and finally it is evident he is going to be successful. The baby's head comes well into view, and the intern grabs a pair of scissors and with two snips of the blades performs an episiotomy, making the outlet of the birth canal larger by incising its outer rim. Within a few seconds, the baby is out, and the intern holds it in one arm as he picks up the bulb syringe with his free hand and suctions the mucous material out of the baby's nose and mouth. Next, he places a clamp across the umbilical cord and cuts the cord in two. The baby begins to cry and the intern passes him to one of the nurses, situating himself again at the foot of the table to deliver the afterbirth, the placenta. He does this by gentle traction on the portion of the cord remaining attached to the placenta. It comes with ease, and all appears well until the intern inspects the episiotomy site. A few choice curse words explode from his mouth as he exclaims: "Call Dr. Harman. Tell him to come right now. I have a laceration into the rectum and need help." The episiotomy has torn into the rectum and left a direct communication between it and the vagina, and now must be sewn in such a way as to close the tear.

By this time, the mother is quiet and resting, the nurses are busy with their duties, and the whole scene is one of anticlimax, except for the intern who is still looking at the episiotomy and shaking his head in disbelief. "Never had it happen before," he says. "I just can't understand it." He keeps repeating those two sentences and says nothing more. All of us are afraid to ask for an explanation of what went wrong or of his plans to redeem the situation; we stand quietly watching. I feel sorry for him. I know it was the mother who had the pain and agony, the mother who went through the process of delivering the baby, and now, the mother who has a tear in her rectum which will have to be closed. It seems only sensible that any feelings ought to be for this poor mother, but somehow the only one I can think of and have any empathy for is the intern who has been through a different type of situation than that experienced by the mother. I somehow sense that he is having the worse experience, has gone through greater mental stress than she. He is obviously affected by this complication, saying very little until the attending staff physician enters the room. The physician is a short, obese man in his mid forties with almost no hair. The town doctors call him "Curly", but this intern addresses him as "Doctor." The patient is soon taken to the operating room where the tear is closed under general anesthesia. Our student world of medicine changes completely once the patient leaves for the operating room. Our world does not yet include total care for the patient. We will not learn how to close a rectal tear or how to treat a patient post-op. On this particular patient our world is a shallow one: We do not have the worry or responsibility for the woman. Instead, we turn to other patients. We are fed the milk problems of obstetrics and gynecology; the meat will come later.

Each of the four in our sub-group is assigned a patient to follow through labor and delivery. I am assigned a mother of four healthy children who is having weak and irregular contractions about every twenty minutes. I am told by the nurse this means she is not near delivery, and I am to sit beside the bed with my hand on her abdomen and record each contraction her uterus makes. She is an obese, jolly, and talkative patient, telling me about her other deliveries, that the first two were born at home, the next two in the hospital. She states the first had been difficult to deliver, but the more babies she had the easier it became. As I sit with one hand on her abdomen, the other propping up my chin, I keep thinking about the woman who just delivered. I know all deliveries can't be that bad, and wonder if she will ever have the desire to have another baby after what she has been through.

Hours pass and the contractions increase to every seven to eight minutes apart, but are still not very forceful. I have used three sheets of paper, writing down the actual time of the contraction, the duration and the strength, using an arbitrary plus one through plus four. Another hour passes and the contractions get stronger and closer together. By three in the morning the nurse tells me the patient is having true labor, and that I should wake the intern to inform him of the progress of the patient if I don't want to deliver the baby in bed. This, I certainly do not want. Neither in bed nor on the delivery table. I was overly eager to deliver a baby the minute I came on the service, but after seeing how difficult delivery can be, it has become the last thing I want to do. I awaken the intern, tell him how close the contractions are, and he gives me instructions to go ahead and get her on the table; he will be right in. This I do, or, I should say, the nurse does while I stand to one side trying to get a gown and gloves on. This is an ordeal in itself. Everything must be sterile from the time I scrub my hands on through the delivery. There is a special way to put on sterile gowns in order not to contaminate them, and a unique way to get the gloves on without touching the outside of them. Presently, I can scrub, gown, and get my gloves on in a correct, orderly fashion, but that's about as far as I know what to do. Only a few hours ago, I watched everything the intern did in getting ready to make the delivery; but now, each small

— 21 —

movement I make seems like a major thought process. Where do I put my hands? I feel awkward standing on both feet—it seems as if I am standing at attention. I don't know what to say to the patient. I smile and nod to her. I have a mask on—she only saw the nod. I wish the intern were here. Only a few hours ago, I watched him go through the "ten easy steps in delivering a baby," but now realize there are at least a thousand steps just getting ready for a delivery. The nurse begins to tell me what to do until the intern arrives; how to drape the patient, where and in what order to place the instruments, and how the umbilical clamp works, and so on.

By this time the patient is having good contractions coming very close together. It is not at all like the previous delivery. She is having some pain but is keeping quiet about it and is not moving all over the table as did the previous patient. The nurse is standing beside her asking what she plans to name the baby.

"This is more like it," I think to myself, still not feeling very sure of myself delivering babies; wishing the intern would come on in—maybe he has fallen back to sleep! I begin to feel apprehension like I've never had before. Do I dare show it by asking the nurse where the intern might be? I ask myself this question three times before the intern sticks his head in the door and stares commandingly. "They just called me to the emergency room. Someone bleeding and they want me quick. You stand there and catch the baby. That's all. Don't try anything special; she's had four already so this one ought to fall out."

"What about an episiotomy?" I inquire, trying to sound at least like I know a little about what is going on.

With that comment, he looks directly at the nurse and says, "I've got to go. Don't let him do anything other than catch the baby and put the umbilical clamp on. I ought to be back by then." He turns and disappears, leaving me the loneliest individual in the world.

I sense I am about to take that giant step toward becoming the doctor I have been thinking so much about. I step right up to the foot of the delivery table and try to act knowledgeable about what I am doing. I can't seem to visualize how to look busy by just standing, waiting for a baby to fall out. I am sure the intern is right and this will be just a routine delivery, that she could deliver at home like her first two; but there again, I am not sure she won't be just like the previous patient and end up in the operating room. I begin to realize why babies are delivered by obstetricians. Nine times out of ten, anyone can deliver a baby by knowing very little, but it is the tenth time that makes all the difference in the world.

I see the little head pushing down. I awkwardly reach out and place an apprehensive hand on the head and let the baby glide into my nervous fingers. I know I am supposed to clamp the umbilical cord, but where did the intern place the clamp? The umbilical cord is two feet long; I don't know where to put the clamp. Does it even matter where? I remember now. I place it adjacent to the umbilicus, suction mucous out of the nose and mouth, and hand the baby to the nurse. The placenta comes with ease. The nurse breaks the silence barrier between us, "I'm giving the Pitressin now, doctor." I am startled at being called a doctor. I decide I have done okay since she used this reference. After all, I do know Pitressin is a drug used to make the uterus squeeze down after delivery, and not many people who are not doctors know that.

"Sure, go ahead," I say confidently. I realize I haven't done much, but I have experienced something new and it is a great feeling. The intern calls to see how things are, and is relieved to hear it was indeed an uneventful delivery. I take a moment to talk to the mother, telling her it was my first delivery. She smiles, and I somehow sense she realizes this is a bigger event for me than it is for her; it is my first, her fifth.

I remove gloves and gown, buy a Coke and pack of cheese crackers out of the machine, and head toward the bed. It is now six A.M. so it takes about three seconds to go to sleep, even with my clothes on.

The new day starts early with only one hour of sleep accomplished. Tonight is an off night and should allow some time to catch up on my rest. Our group meets in the residents' lounge and decides who has to draw blood from the patients. The only fair way is to rotate four at a time, and since we already have a schedule for who will be on call each night, we decide to let the students draw blood the next morning. All that means to me is that I am supposed to go draw blood. I have never stuck a needle into anything; yet, I am now required to stick every patient on the floor for blood. I have to remind myself of the rule I discovered taking those courses which weren't too interesting only a year ago: I must discipline myself to do things I don't like in order to achieve my major goal which in turn will reward me for my work. Okay, it worked in those courses, it can work now. I do not like walking up to a person and causing him pain while I learn to stick needles into veins. Yet, I must accomplish this by immediate action. RIGHT NOW!

I muster up courage and walk into the room of the first patient I am to "stick." I explain my mission as best I can to the patient as I place a tourniquet around her arm. My conversation sounds as if I were reading my sentences. I stick the needle through the skin on top of a vein in plain view just below the tourniquet. The needle slides to the side of the vein. I withdraw and try again. I finally get the needle through the skin and into the vein with the patient leaning closer and closer to my face. I glance up at her with a slight smile and say, "You really have hard veins to hit." She replies that they were not that hard to hit yesterday, and that no one else had this much trouble getting blood from her. I can't bring myself to tell her that the student who drew blood just the morning before had a year's experience while I am having my first try.

I withdraw enough blood to fill one test tube. I have to fill two tubes, but can't withdraw any more blood. Evidently, the needle has slipped out of the veins. I withdraw the needle and hold pressure over the site, but blood continues to come out of the needle hole.

The patient starts wiggling her fingers. "That tourniquet is hurting my arm and making my hand tingle."

How stupid can I be? Obviously the vein will keep building up pressure and bleed as long as the tourniquet is on. I take it off, and the bleeding stops. My big worry now is to get the other test tube of blood. No one has ever mentioned all the major problems that go with learning to become a doctor. This is all assumed until it presents itself for the first time. I have one tube of blood and need another, I don't want to see this patient again in my life, much less stick her again. I am sure the feeling its mutual. I walk out into the hall and meet a fellow student who is waiting for me. He was unable to get any blood at all from his patient, and wants me to try my luck. It suddenly dawns on me that my problem is solved. After all, I have drawn one tube of blood from my patient; he ought to be able to draw one. We agree to swap patients and try again.

I walk into the room of the patient my friend attempted to stick. "Are you any better than the last doctor that was in here?"

"Well, I've had a little more experience," I reply. I am honest. I have drawn blood, he hasn't.

We both are successful due to some unknown fate, but I decide right away that I am not going to take any blood drawing rotation every fourth morning. I am going to be here *every* morning until I can draw blood from any patient I try. I glance at the *Goal's Rule Book* from time to time just as a reminder. Immediate action—there is no problem with that. There are few minutes in the day when I am not actively working on my goal on O.B. With a subject this interesting, I don't have to work so hard in making myself stick to the rules.

As the rotation progresses, I begin to hit the majority of veins I attempt—one hurdle passed. I am delivering babies with some regularity and do not feel out of place standing at the foot of the delivery table. The excitement and newness of the first clinical rotation wears down as the clerkship draws to an end. I have enjoyed O.B., but I don't think I want to do this for the rest of my life. I refuel my eagerness to learn something new and make ready to move on to the next rotation—pediatrics.

I review my goal's book and bring it up to date, something I have started doing from time to time. MAJOR: Surgeon; INTERMEDIATE: Medical school; IMMEDIATE ACTION: Study pediatrics—RIGHT NOW. Don't wade into it for a week or two, get aggressive now and learn all that is possible on the first day. I am learning more and more that immediate action is the key to successfully reaching a major goal. What I do right now determines what the outcome will eventually be. The price is paid *now*.

As I think of goals, I think of Harriet and our achieved goal of marriage. Harriet is an ideal wife. She is teaching the second grade at a school near our apartment. We are living on her salary alone, and the meals reflect this perfectly.

"Sweetie, do you realize I have now eaten tuna fish fixed thirty-eight different ways?" I remark as I dish up a big spoonful of tuna casserole onto my plate.

"I only fixed it because you complained about the Spam last night," is her brisk reply.

We have been married just long enough for me to develop a sense about her. My sense tells me I have said enough. In fact, I have probably said too much. I will be glad when next year comes, and she gets a raise. She does do a good job with tuna fish. For this I am thankful.

Life as a married man and a maturing third year student continues. I begin the new rotation of pediatrics, and after only two days of orientation I can see that it is completely different from the O.B. rotation. The diseases, diagnosis, medication, and treatment are all on a much different scale from that of an adult. After the first few days of ward duty, I become somewhat discouraged with working with infants. Unlike adult patients, they cannot tell me, or show me, where they hurt, and I can't seem to find where they hurt by direct examination because they usually cry from the time I begin the exam until I quit. I had a difficult enough time memorizing the dosages of adult medicine on O.B., and now this mental process has to be redone but on a much more accurate basis since a small difference in the dose makes a big difference to a small child or infant.

The rotation begins at the university hospital, and I am placed on a team of doctors consisting of a staff man, a senior resident, a junior resident, an intern, and four students. I am assigned to Tom Moore, the junior resident, and am to take orders from him. We make rounds and attend conferences in the mornings, hold clinics in the afternoon. Students are required to remain at the hospital every third night to be on call, which consists of being called initially if something happens to one of the patients on the floor. After seeing the patient, the student decides whether he can handle the situation or needs to call an intern. The intern does likewise, and he is responsible to the first year resident, and so on it goes up the ladder until, on a complicated case, the whole team will be present seeing the patient. I soon realize that the whole basis for medical teaching has to be this chain of command, and there is no cut and dried method of knowing where the chain stops. One first year resident may be able to handle a situation superbly while his fellow first year resident may have no idea what is going on, necessitating aid from the second year man. The one lesson I do learn having to rotate at night with this type of set-up is: If there is any doubt whatsoever as to the proper treatment of the patient—call the next higher man. This does three things: There is more assurance that the patient is treated correctly, it transfers the responsibility from me to someone more responsible, and it presents the opportunity to learn from someone with more experience. After trying this chain of command a few times, I begin to understand an important fact of life. There are basically two ways to learn anything. One is by direct experience, and the other is by being smart enough to benefit from the experiences of others. On the one hand, there is the "I have to go through myself" experience, and on the other hand the "I don't have to go through myself" experience. Medical training is set up for me to learn directly from the individual above me in the "chain." I shouldn't have to make the same mistakes or go through the same experiences just to learn what he knows. If I am smart, I will observe him and ask as many questions as I can pump to him to keep from having to re-enact everything he has done wrong. I reason one step further. If I am really smart, I will look ahead to the entire chain above me and tuck away in my mind some of their experiences, even though I am not far enough along to have a direct benefit from them at this time. I will form a small storehouse of these "I don't have to go through myself" experiences for future reference. If possible, I will learn as much as I can through other people's experiences. I will try to learn as many "I don't have to go through myself" experiences as possible on these clinical rotations. The patients won't have to suffer, and I will learn.

Dr. Keith Milton is the chairman of the pediatrics department and closely simulates a whirlwind in everything he does. The entire staff likes and respects him, but there are very few students or residents who don't get reprimanded by him at least twice. He is everywhere at once, on rounds one minute, in a conference the next, and grabbing me by the arm to go see an interesting patient the next.

By the fifth night on call, I feel comfortable on the service. The awkwardness of being a new student on a new rotation has vanished; I know the patients and some of the treatments. All is quiet until I am awakened by an intruder in our sleeping quarters. The lights go on. Someone is stomping around the room yelling, "Let's go! I don't have all night to pussyfoot around. I've got to fly to Chicago in the morning, and I want to see how the patients are doing." I rise up in bed, look at my watch. It is two-thirty A.M. All of a sudden I realize Dr. Milton is the originator of the talking. He has been out of town for three days and his plane has just come in.

"This fellow must be crazy," I think. "He hasn't even been home, and now he wants to make rounds in the middle of the night." I drag out of bed feeling sure it won't take long to make rounds since we have very few sick patients on the ward.

I am proven wrong. We finish rounds at five o'clock, and the intern has five or six items to be ordered on each patient. These are things even Tom, the resident, had not thought of, much less told us to do.

Dr. Milton takes off to the nurses station, pours each of us a cup of coffee and starts talking. At least it is a nice gesture to pour our coffee, and apparently he is going to become more informal, possibly talk about his recent trip. I am ready for a few minutes of discussing something other than patients.

Instead, he says, "I don't ever want to leave town and come back with the pediatric service looking the way it does now. Tom, I'll see you when I get back. Now, let's get to work." And with that verbal order, he is off down the hall and gone for another week. We all sit calmly drinking our coffee, saying very little. It is difficult to believe the preceding events actually happened. All the responsibility lay on Tom's shoulders even though many of the things that did not get done, and many of the laboratory results which were not memorized, were not his fault, but that of the intern and me. There is nothing I would rather do than return to bed, but I know I won't even *see* the bed until I am home after another full day. We are too far behind on our work to think of a nap now.

The weeks pass. Often during this portion of my pediatric rotation, I have caught myself becoming annoyed with Dr. Milton's dictatorial, authoritative role in running the service. Only as I near the completion of working with him do I realize the fantastic amount of knowledge I have learned from this man and his unique form of teaching. He *makes* his students learn. He doesn't leave it to the prerogative of the student to read his assignment, depending on whether he has time or wants to. He will ask questions on the subjects he expects us to know. I regret that I realize only now how great a teacher he is. I could have learned more from him initially if I had the respect for him then that I do now. Dr. Milton's goal makes him the way he is. His goal is to have the best possible pediatric department. His goal is not to be the best liked professor on the staff, because the two goals are not in harmony. He can't be very well liked if he wakes us in the middle of the night and keeps us up the rest of the night. But, it just may be the reason he has one of the best pediatric departments in the country. The goal makes the man's character what it is. I pledge to surround myself with teachers like Dr. Milton in the future if at all possible.

I try to think more about what it is that makes Dr. Milton so successful in his field of medicine. What makes him the Chief? What sets him above everyone else in the department? If I can figure that out, then I can decide how to conduct my activities accordingly. I first rehash in my mind what I have already put together and see if there is anything to add to the picture of attaining goals—my goals. One thing—he has made a habit of doing things the other staff men don't like to do. He has made a habit of working at any time of the day or night, because there may not be any other time for his work. The other staff men would rather be at home in bed asleep. He has repeated this work habit so long, it has become a part of his character. So, I should be able to determine my work character by deciding to do things the other students don't particularly like to do and continue to do it until it becomes a habit. His life is one big habit. He doesn't have to stop and think about how he is going to handle rounds. It is automatic. It is a habit to him.

I turn a few pages over in my *Goal's Rule Book* and write the word: CHARACTER: Summation of one's habits. HABIT: Repetition of immediate actions.

Also, Dr. Milton is persistent in his character. There is no question in my mind exactly where he stands when it comes to care for his patients. It has to be right—black or white, clear-cut—right. I add a new word to the list on the "Thoughts" page in the back of the *Goal's Rule Book*. That word is PERSISTENCE: A necessary ingredient to success.

Immediate actions, persistence, habit, character. These form a logical plan to build goals on. I will try to remember these as I continue through the rotation which consists of Pinewood Hospital and the nursery. Tomorrow, I start at Pinewood, which is a state institution for mentally retarded children.

I have read extensively about retarded children and have quickly grown to dislike looking at the terrible pictures I see in the textbook. After beginning rounds the first morning, it takes only minutes to realize that the actual patients are ten times worse than what is written. After ten minutes, I am ready to go back and ask for an extended rotation with Dr. Milton. These grotesque figures of human anatomy send the eye searching, but at the same time make one try to block out from one's mind what it is actually seeing. There is nothing proud, nothing ambitious about these children. They will not have goals nor master habits. These children are not like the ones seen on television in campaigns for the mentally retarded; these are the ones only a fraction of civilization ever sees. There is one four-year-old child who has a head as large as a basketball. During his waking hours he only sits and stares. Another child is tied with a sheet in a chair while he makes uncoordinated movements with his arms and head, saliva drooling off his chin onto his chest.

After being at Pinewood only ten hours, I am more depressed than at any other time since starting school. All these helpless children, so little to do to help them. I am glad there are doctors who are interested enough and dedicated enough to spend their lives studying and treating these children, for I know I don't possess what it takes to practice this type of medicine.

I elect to avoid this ward of the hospital in the future; I cannot control my mind enough to cope with such problems. I know I should be able to, but as yet I have not found a way. I flip through what I have written in my goal's book, but cannot come up with a convincing argument that it is necessary to dwell on these patients in order to become a surgeon.

There are patients in another section of the hospital who can function adequately in the institution's environment. These are children with low IQs—many very pleasant and affectionate. These are the ones I have seen in public and on television running in the "Olympics for the Retarded." These I can envision being helped enough to make their own way in society. I see many in this ward exerting more effort to accomplish something than ninety percent of the "normal" population do. Perhaps we could learn more about accomplishing goals from these patients than from successful people in the "real" world.

I begin spending more and more time with these patients looking for some insight to better understand what makes them go. Why do they try so hard? What is their secret? I am aware they are the less endowed ones; yet, I think they may have something that the rest of us don't have and could use. I spend some of my thought time at night trying to solve the riddle of what drives them so hard. Obviously, they cannot think of a multitude of goals at any one time. They can't learn to ride a bicycle, shoot a basketball, play dodgeball, and dress themselves completely all in the same day. Yet, there are some riding bicycles, others shooting basketballs, and others very proud they have buttoned their own sweaters correctly. If there is something to learn from them, it lies in the fact that they go at things one step at a time. They don't sit down and plan to learn to dress by themselves, or ride a bicycle to the playground, or play basketball. But there are some of them who first learned to dress, then learned to ride a bicycle, and then learned to shoot a basketball. The entire sequence could have been too much of an undertaking; one step at a time was not. One step at a time seems the answer to their major accomplishments.

I write in my book for future reference: ONE STEP AT A TIME —The path to accomplishment of goals. I have just proved I can learn even from these children.

I soon become accustomed to being around the retarded. I say accustomed because I felt like an outsider invading the privacy of these children's lives when I first arrived, and it has taken over a week for me to accept this institution. The children had no adjusting in accepting me; the adjusting has been all on my part. Unilateral—that is the irony of it all; I am learning from them!

There are several adults who have been here since childhood, and many of these are the most interesting to observe. There is one patient who is about thirty years old. Even though his IQ is low and he can't read, write, or take care of himself, he has the unusual ability to know what time it is within two minutes of the correct time without looking at a clock; he doesn't even have a watch. "Fool John" is the only name I have ever heard him called. Everytime I see him, I always ask him the time and he is always correct. I wonder how he does this so precisely. I see him standing alone in the hall looking out the window. I decide to ask him directly how he can do this. Maybe he will tell me some great secret he has not told anyone else. I ask him how he does it. He smiles, makes a motion like he is winding a watch on his forehead and replies, "I have a clock inside my head and I keep it wound all the time." I watch as he walks off down the hall making the same winding motion on his ear, his chin, and his nose. It is fascinating to believe someone like John can pull this ingenuous feat time and again. There is much more about the mind we don't know, especially John's mind.

This happens to be my night on call and it turns out to be a workless evening. I read a while and drop off to sleep, only to be awakened by the ringing of the phone. The nurse on the line says there is a boy, six years old, with a temperature of 101 degrees, and she wants me to check him. I dress, walk to the next building, and go through the usual examination of his ears, throat, neck, and lungs and find nothing to explain the fever. I don't want to start antibiotics without locating a source of infection, so I know I need to find some reason for the fever.

The nurse senses my bewilderment. "Doctor, do you think he could have a fecal impaction? That causes a high fever in these children lots of times."

I perceive this as a nice way of her telling me to do a rectal examination and check for an impaction. Sure enough, he is impacted. Looking at his chart, I find he has not had a bowel movement for five days. I order enemas and laxatives, and after performing the messy chore of cleaning out his rectum, return to my room. Usually I don't have any trouble going back to sleep after getting up in the middle of the night, but occasionally I return to bed and my mind stays awake no matter how much I want to sleep. It brings up the awareness of my next test. I don't want to even think about that, and let the thought fade into darkness. But now, another thought creeps to the forefront of my mind: "Fool John." "Fool John." "Fool John." The more I think about John and his strange ability to tell time, the more I wonder if his ability is functional in the middle of the night. I know I can look at my watch in the morning, and if I keep up with the time throughout the day, I can guess fairly close to the correct time. I think perhaps this is what John does. I have thought that all along, but there is only one sure way to find out.

I get up again, dress, walk over to building number three where John rooms. I slip quietly through the main lobby, past the nurse's desk, and on down the hall to his room. I ease the door open and walk to his bed. "John . . John," I whisper, as I shake his shoulder. "What time is it?"

John doesn't move an inch, but only opens his eyes at the same time his customary smile appears on his lips. "Twenty-five after three," he whispers back and then shuts his eyes. He is still smiling when I leave his bedside. As I walk toward my on-call room, I know John must feel some sense of superiority, making me get out of bed in the middle of the night to ask him what time it is. I wonder how many other students have tried to "fool" John. I get back in bed at three-thirty and actually glance at my watch to check the time. For some reason, I feel foolish as I realize I'm looking at my watch only five minutes after "Fool John" told me the correct time.

I finish the rotation at Pinewood Hospital almost in disbelief that there are so many normal, well-formed children in the world. After being here only three weeks, I am almost afraid to try to have a family. I have never known before there are so many possibilities of a malformed or retarded infant being born. Very few realize how blessed it is to have normal children. Perhaps it is best for most not to know of the possibilities. From one viewpoint I wish I were ignorant of the facts, but this portion of my medical education has been enlightening, although depressing.

During my rotation at Pinewood, I have tried to tell Harriet of what I've seen. However, she seems to be content to remain ignorant of the facts.

"I don't want to hear about it," Harriet cuts me off as I start to recount my rotation with the mentally retarded. She is preparing for tomorrow's class, and I am taking a little break from my reading.

"I don't think just talking about it will have any effect on whether we have a mentally retarded baby or not," I reply, trying to get her to put her books down and talk to me a minute.

"I don't want to talk about it!" She never even gives me a glance.

"When do you want to start planning a family?" This question catches her off guard and causes her to immediately put her books down. She looks up and smiles.

"I don't know. I would like to be able to stay home with the baby whenever we do have one. So, I guess that puts it just after you start internship. You will make a small salary, I can quit teaching and we can start having our children. I will stay home and cook you something more than creamed tuna on toast." Harriet comes over and sits down on my lap. She likes to talk about the children we will someday have. I think she is going to make a good mother.

With my rotation over at Pinewood, I return to the medical center to complete the pediatric rotation. However, I have mixed emotions. Though I have left the physical location of Pinewood and tried to leave the memory of the first ward I visited behind, I find it is stamped on my mind forever.

This last portion of pediatrics rotation will be spent in the nursery, which requires being present at all deliveries, checking the infants initially, and carrying them to the nursery. We are taught to examine the newborn and give them a rating in proportion to how good their reflexes are, their color, and their general response.

It feels good to be back under Dr. Milton's wing, even though the work load will be ten times greater than at Pinewood. Pinewood was one of those experiences you have to learn firsthand. No one can quite tell you what it is like. It is an "I have to go through myself" experience. Dr. Milton is a great one to learn from, especially the "I don't have to go through myself" situations. He doesn't mind telling you the things that have not worked for him. And he is quick to tell you they won't work for you either.

We walk into the lecture room a few doors down from the nursery to attend his first lecture on "The Care of the Nursery Infant." Dr. Milton clears his throat and begins: "On certain occasions a newborn does not breathe properly, so the pediatrician has to place a tube through his mouth and into the windpipe and breathe for him. This consists of putting a laryngoscope, which is like a small tongue blade with a light on the end, into the infant's mouth to visualize the back of the throat and on down the windpipe. Next, a hollow rubber tube about half the size of a pencil is placed through the mouth and down the larynx." Dr. Milton picks up a laryngoscope and an endotracheal tube and holds them for all to see. He walks over to a small oxygen tank and continues his lecture. "Oxygen can then be delivered directly to the lungs by connecting the oxygen to this bag that fits onto the rubber tubing. You can breathe for the infant. This is like mouth-to-mouth respiration except there is a direct tube to the lungs and a bag is used for the ventilating process. This can be a life-saving procedure, but you have to remember the most critical point of the entire situation is the time factor. You are working with a very small baby, with very small instruments, and under a life or death situation, the outcome depends on whether the tube can be placed correctly and quickly." He pauses for effect, and then as he turns toward us, he drops everything he is holding. All of us jump and shift in our chairs as we watch the instruments bounce as they hit the floor. Now that he has everyone's attention, he continues. "Some day you will be the only one around to put the tube down an infant's windpipe. Will you be able to do it, or will you try unsuccessfully and see the infant die? Think about that." His eyes shift from one student to another until he has "contacted" every student present. "I want every one of you to be able to intubate a newborn infant by the time you leave my service. The first infant born dead, day or night, I want the entire group to be called in and each of you to take your turn passing the tube until you can do it on the first try, five times in a row."

My immediate reaction is how inhumane it seems. I attempt to switch my mind from that of a layman to that of a physician. As a "layman medical student," I think of the poor, innocent infant who has come into the world without life or breath. I have to concentrate awhile before I express my displeasure at intubating a dead infant. I make myself look ahead to the next time an infant is born who may need intubation. I know Dr. Milton is correct and accept his reasoning, knowing it is something I must learn to perform even though it will be difficult to do. I think back on one of my rules—I must go ahead and do what I don't want to do in order to reach my goal. If I do only what I *want* to do, I will never learn to intubate a baby. After all, I surely would not want to be passing a tube at a critical time without ever having practiced at a non-critical time. When that situation really does occur and no one else is around with any experience in intubation, the infant may survive only because I know how to do the job correctly and quickly by previous practice on a dead baby. Call it rationalization, call it whatever, but I convince myself to do it and furthermore, I am convinced it is the right thing to do.

Our first stillborn comes in the middle of the night, and we are called in from home. Sleepily, I drive to the hospital and climb the stairs to the nursery. Within the next few minutes, our entire group of eight students is all present and the resident goes through the procedure of intubation step by step, insuring that each of us knows what to do. Then he leaves us with a dead infant, a laryngoscope, and several endotracheal tubes of varying sizes. One by one, we start to practice passing the tube. My turn comes, it looked easy enough for the resident, but I can't find the epiglottis, the beginning of the windpipe. Within the next thirty minutes, the worth of this night exercise becomes very evident. I can see myself trying to do this on an infant in distress without having done it in practice many times before. We practice until proficiency is obtained and by the time we are through, each of us can intubate in less than six seconds from the time we pick up the instrument to the time we connect the breathing bag to the tube.

I drive home in the chilly morning air with a feeling of accomplishment and know at last I have learned something which gives me the ability to save a life in a situation in which perhaps no one else can help. This is the first time I have ever experienced this feeling, and in these early morning hours I have a small taste of what becoming a doctor is all about. Some of the immediate goals of action are beginning to pay off, and for the first time I get a fleeting taste of what my intermediate goal tastes like—being a real doctor. Not only that, but I am also realizing that the "I have to go through myself" experiences are the most difficult experiences and that no one could teach them to me. They are absolutely necessary even though I don't relish going through them. If I am to ever be successful, I must, I must, I must go ahead and do the necessary things I don't want to do. That is a point. These are things no one else likes to do; most won't do them. Few do them, but these few will reach the goal successfully.

I finish pediatrics learning much about the practice of pediatrics plus learning much about goals. With these thoughts implanted, I begin the rotation I waited two and a half years to start—general surgery. I look to surgery as having all the excitement I will ever want to deal with in everyday work. There also seems to be some intangible significance of actually doing something with your hands rather than just prescribing medicine for the patient. At last, I get to find out—firsthand.

My first day of surgery begins by reporting to the ward and meeting with the residents. The chief resident is the "big gun" who calls all the shots since he has the most experience on the team. Our chief resident is Ben Harris. He is pleasant and easygoing, but best of all he likes to teach. Formal lectures are given by the attending staff each day, but much of the practical teaching is done by the residents. Ben greets us and introduces the rest of the team consisting of a third year resident, a second year resident, a first year resident and two interns.

While making rounds the first morning, it appears that there is a definite pattern concerning which resident performs which operation. The first patient on rounds is a man who was admitted to the hospital because of poor circulation to his leg. An above-the-knee amputation, called an "A-K" amputation by the intern presenting the patient to us, has been performed. This is an "intern case" meaning it is easy enough so that someone just starting in surgical training can handle the procedure. Other intern cases we see on the rounds include an appendectomy, a hemorrhoidectomy, and a split thickness skin graft where a thin piece of skin has been taken off a burn patient's thigh and placed on the site of the burn, his chest.

The first year residents make formal presentations of their patients to us and these operations seem to be a little more difficult than the intern cases. There are several hernias, a patient who has had a V-shaped wedge removed from his lower lip in order to excise a small cancer, and several similar types of cases which seemingly could be done by either the intern or the first year resident, depending on whether or not the first year man would give the case to the intern.

The second year resident presents a huge woman with gall bladder disease. The resident removes the dressing and notices the wound is red and swollen. He takes out some of the stitches, which results in foul smelling pus pouring out between the skin edges and down the side of her abdomen. He grabs a handful of gauze pads from the dressing tray and tries to catch as much of it as he can without getting it all over the patients's abdomen. "I knew she was too fat not to get infected." He appears angry as he slaps a dressing over the now open wound. His anger melts into an understanding smile as he looks up at the horrified patient. "That will be a couple of weeks healing, but it will be okay. It just means we'll have to clean it several times a day, and show you how to take care of it. In a few days I think you will be able to clean it at home and get out of the hospital on time."

The patient lies there nodding her head and staring at the dressing. I am about as horrified as she is. I have never seen an infected wound drained before and am sure the patient has not witnessed such a sight herself, much less experienced it. It looks awful. I think it should merit much more than a brief comment from the resident in assuring the patient, and me, that the infected wound is going to heal rather than fall apart and allow all her intestines to protrude through the wound. I will accept his statement for the time being, but plan to watch the wound daily to see exactly how quickly it heals or whether the intestines actually will come falling out. I guess this situation is just like everything else in life. What is common to one is assumed to be common to all. The first time this resident had one of his patients with a wound infection, he probably spent an extra hour reassuring the patient, convincing her it would be all right. But after seeing several infections and seeing them all heal, he forgets that his knowledge is one-sided, that the patient has not had the privilege of seeing ten infected wounds heal.

The same resident next presents a woman from whom he has removed a lobe of the thyroid gland in which he used a subcuticular stitch to close the incision. He points out that the stitches were placed just under the skin and would be absorbed by the body; no stitches are visible on the skin. This closure has been done so nicely and meticulously that even now the incision can hardly be seen. I can tell he is proud of the closure because he jokingly asks one of the students if he can detect where the patient was operated on.

The most difficult and spectacular cases are performed by the chief resident. He has had more experience than anyone on the team and has to take the responsibility, not only for his patients, but all the cases done on the entire service. He walks into the room of a patient who looks like he has lost half his face. Ben places his hand on the patient's shoulder and addresses us: "This man had a 'commando' procedure. We call it that because after the operation it looks like a commando dropped a grenade on his face and then expected us to close the wound. He had cancer on the floor of his mouth which we resected along with his mandible, and a radical neck dissection on the same side. That means resecting his jaw bone and all the lymph nodes and fat tissue in the neck from the collarbone up to the jaw." Ben looks at the student standing beside me. "I want you to be able to tell me the chances this man has of being cured. As a matter of fact, you can discuss cancer of the floor of the mouth on rounds tomorrow afternoon." Turning to the patient he says, "I think your chances are good myself, but let's see what our new student has to say." And with that we are off to the next room.

Ben introduces the patient as we gather around his bed. "Mr. Smallwood had a blockage of his superficial femoral artery, one of the main arteries in the thigh, and was developing what we call intermittent claudication. He could walk only about a block and then would have to stop to rest because there was not enough blood getting to his leg. This made the calf muscles cramp. Intermittently, he would stop to rest and allow enough circulation to return to enable him to walk another block before the pain hit again. I did a femoral arteriogram on him. For those who flunked radiology, this means I injected dye, which will show up on x-ray, into the main artery in the thigh and could then outline the block inside the artery very nicely. We will go over those films in x-ray conference this afternoon. Anyway, I put in a bypass graft, which is a cloth tube sewn above and below the block in the artery which diverts the blood through the tube and around the blockage. You can now feel his posterior tibial pulse—his ankle pulse—which means there is an adequate blood flow resulting in a pain free leg."

This time he points to me: "I want you to look up the symptoms and progression of peripheral vascular diseases and be able to explain them in detail by tomorrow."

Ben steps to the next bed and looks at Bart Moore, probably the most intelligent student in our group. "This patient had surgery for a duodenal ulcer. Do you know anything about ulcers?"

"Yes, I have read about them," he replies confidently.

"What percent of patients can be treated medically?"

"I'm not sure. Most of them."

"Eighty-five percent. What percent are *cured* with medicines?"

"Most of them."

"Wrong. Only five percent become asymptomatic with no recurrence of symptoms. What are the indications for surgery?"

"Bleeding, perforation, obstruction . . ." Bart answers without hesitation. He had memorized these indications straight out of the textbook just for this moment as if he knew Ben was going to ask that very question. In all of medical school, I have never had that set of circumstances happen to me; if I know the answer, I am not asked the question.

Ben finishes Bart's answer, ". . . and unsuccessful medical management. There are four indications, but I guess three out of four isn't bad." Ben realizes he is questioning one of the smarter ones in the class and uses him to teach the rest of us. "Okay, now you have decided to operate. What procedure are you going to perform?"

"A vagotomy—cutting the nerves to the stomach and pyloroplasty."

"What does a vagotomy do?"

"Decreases the acid secretion of the stomach."

"What is pyloroplasty?"

"I am not sure just how you do it, but it enlarges the outlet of the stomach. That also decreases the amount of acid in the stomach."

"What other operation could you perform?"

"A vagotomy and antrectomy."

"How does that differ from a vagotomy and pyloroplasty?

"The bottom portion of the stomach is removed."

"Dr. Moore," Ben addresses the not-yet doctor, "I hope you realize you have only scratched the surface of knowledge about peptic ulcer disease. Before you leave the service, I hope we can teach you the thorough physiology behind all your answers." Ben heads for the next room.

I hate to be put on the spot like Bart just was, but I have come to realize that that is the best way to retain knowledge—to actually be the one called on in class to discuss a subject. A poor second best, I have concluded, is to be the spectator at such a session. Worse yet is to try to learn it from a book. At the beginning of medical school, I thought learning from a book was the only source of knowledge, but I am coming to learn that facts on the pages are only the first layer of cement and steel in the foundation of a skyscraper. This situation relates back to the two basic sources of experience I learned at Pinewood Institution. The "I don't have to go through myself" type is beneficial, but relates to being the observer in this situation. The "I have to go through myself" experience Bart just went through is the most traumatic, but is also the most rewarding in remembering a subject for the future.

As I follow our group to the next patient, I begin to realize that there is something distinctively different about the surgical residents from residents on the other services. For one thing, morning rounds begin at six-thirty instead of the usual eight o'clock. There is always something to do either in the operating room or with the patients on the floor—dressings to be changed, wounds to be cleaned, burn patients to be continuously taken care of, post operative checks on seriously ill patients. This is truly a working service that never stops.

Also, the lesson learned from the children at Pinewood begins to fit here at the medical center. The children learned to button their sweaters and coats. The intern learns to do an appendectomy. The children next learned to ride a bicycle. The first year resident learns to do a hernia. The children learned to dribble a basketball. The second year resident learns to perform stomach surgery. And finally, the children could get up, dress themselves, get on a bicycle, ride to the playground, and play a game of basketball. Whereas finally, the intern becomes resident, then chief resident, putting all his skills together to do it all. The same chief resident was once an intern who had to complete one immediate action goal at a time to achieve a successful year at internship to go on to complete his intermediate goal of junior resident to fulfill his major goal of chief residency and becoming a complete surgeon.

Speaking of immediate action goals, I need to get over to the library to study peripheral vascular diseases as soon as I can find time. Immediate goal for the moment: Read all I can on peripheral vascular disease *today*.

When we finally finish evening rounds at six-thirty, I waste no time heading straight for the library to study my assignment for tomorrow. I am elated, think I could study surgery all night for sheer enjoyment. There is so much to learn and I need to begin building my storehouse of knowledge. By midnight, I realize how little I know about vascular diseases and how much more reading I will have to do by tomorrow afternoon to be able to discuss it. I roll into bed at one A.M. thinking back over the first day on surgery and can't go to sleep. I have the same kind of excitement I used to get on Christmas Eve or the night before going on a trip. Four years of college, almost three years of medical school, and at last, I am studying what I have thought so much about: surgery.

Harriet senses my excitement as I keep her awake talking about how busy we're going to be on surgery. She doesn't say much, just lies in bed staring at the ceiling, listening. After ten minutes of my chattering, she leans over and gives me a kiss on my cheek telling me I had better go to sleep or I won't feel like getting up in the morning. However, I lay awake long after I hear her breathing deeply in slumber. It's going to be fun to be a surgeon.

My excitement carries over to the following morning as I awake easily. I beat the residents to the hospital for six-thirty rounds. Today is an operating day for "our" team, and I am scheduled to scrub with Ben on a patient with cancer of the colon. I am listed as third assistant, which means there will be Ben, a first year resident, an intern, and then myself to scrub on the case. "First surgeon" carries the same connotation as being labeled "president of the corporation." The surgeon given this title is in complete command at the operating table; whatever he says is final. He takes full responsibility for the patient and everyone else is subordinate. I am listed as third assistant and must work my way up the ladder of surgical study and expertise until I am listed as first surgeon. Even when Ben has the chairman of the department scrubbing on a case with him, he is still listed as first surgeon and assumes the first responsibility for the patient. If anything goes wrong with the case, it is the first surgeon who explains the situation to the patient's family, the first surgeon who takes the credit for the case, whether it be successful or a failure. It is not a label given without forethought and deserving credit, and is not received without the self-assurance required to perform the particular procedure. One of the more senior residents recently dropped out of the surgery program solely because he was not willing to take the responsibility that coincides with being first surgeon.

After rounds, I change into a scrub suit and follow the intern into the operating room. Ben makes a midline incision in the lower abdomen and soon is packing the intestines out of the way by covering them with a moist towel. He places two metal retractors on top of the towel and turns to me. "Now's your big chance to get in on some surgery. Hold these." Two and a half hours later I am still holding them. I admit this isn't a very large part of the overall procedure, but at least I have a front row seat to what is going on. Plus the fact that I feel just as successful right now doing what I am doing as Ben does performing the operation. I feel this way because I can see myself as a surgeon, just as Ben is. I don't actually possess these qualities, but there is no doubt in my mind that someday I will possess them. Therefore, I can have a similar feeling of success being third assistant as I will have when I become chief resident. I realize I have been successful as long as I have been working toward my major goal, but this is the first time I have really felt the successful feeling. I am actually standing at an operating table working on a real live patient. My mind will let me begin to put it all together and see the real possibility of what it will be like. I have reached a milestone—tangible reality that I can actually become a chief resident.

My mind shifts from what I am doing and I relax on the retractors only two seconds, but the intestines begin to slip around the retractor blades and fall down into the operative field. I am not sure what to do. All he said was to hold the retractor, which I am doing. Ben stops, replaces the intestines behind the retractors, and speaks to me without lifting his eyes from the operative field. "You've got to keep looking. If you can't see, I can't see. And if I can't see, I can't do the operation. And if I can't do the operation there's no use in your being here, so keep those guts out of the way." I nod and continue my grip on the retractors. He does an excellent job getting the cancer out and the large bowel reconnected.

He starts the closure by placing a large suture through the tough fascia layer of the abdomen. "This is what holds the wound together," Ben states. This fascia layer and nothing else." He looks up at me. "You thought the skin held the incision together, didn't you?"

"I thought it helped."

"Nope. Sewing the skin together just makes the skin edges grow properly. This deep fascia layer is the one that does the job. This is the important layer—the layer the patient can't see. The patient judges the whole operation by the way the skin is put together and that is the least important part of the procedure." By now Ben is almost ready to start closing the skin.

"Do you know how to sew skin?" Ben delays starting his sewing and looks directly at me.

"Yes. I have never closed skin in an operation, but I know how it is done." I see a chance to get to do some operating, even if it is only to close the skin; the most important part of the procedure according to the patient.

Ben hands me the needle holder and tissue pickups. I feel awkward. I feel that everything in the room has stopped, and everyone is watching me. I start sewing, but my hands don't seem to want to do what my mind tells them to do. They work as stiff as chopsticks. My shoulders are the only joints that want to try to coordinate my hand movements. My elbows, wrists, and fingers are frozen. It is as if my two hands were connected to two separate people rather than both being fed by one central nervous system. It looked so easy when Ben was holding the instruments. Finally, I manage to get the incision closed and hope the patient realizes how insignificant the skin closure is in this operation.

As soon as the case is over, Ben takes me to the resident's lounge and explains what he did in surgery. He discusses cancer of the colon, goes over the prognosis, the symptoms the patient usually presents to the doctor, and how much bowel to resect. This fifteen minutes of individual lecturing makes the entire morning worthwhile. Much of medical learning is done in this way. Yesterday, Ben could have spent the same fifteen minutes telling me about cancer of the colon, and by today I would not recall ten percent of the knowledge he taught me. However, standing at the operating table for three hours watching the cancer being removed, watching a patient being cured before my eyes, enables my brain to make an impressive recording of what Ben tells me in fifteen minutes, and I will be able to recall ninety percent of it tomorrow. Not only that, but I will be able to use that ninety percent as a base for further information to be built upon. Even though it appeared to be much wasted time while I stood at the operating table holding retractors, this time was used very efficiently in preparing my mind for knowledge of cancer of the colon, which will be useful to me the rest of my surgical life.

My mind races back to something I thought at the operating table: "I can see myself already as a surgeon, just as much as Ben is . . . I can have a similar feeling of success." As long as I am working toward becoming a surgeon, I will have this feeling of success. In my own mind, I will be successful as long as I am working *toward* the goal of becoming a surgeon. I add this to the *Goal's Rule Book*: SUCCESS: I am successful as long as I am working toward my major goal. I don't have to wait until I actually complete surgical training to be successful. I am a success *now*! (As a matter of fact, I became a success that day in high school when I decided to become a doctor and began working toward that goal.)

I had better get on with some immediate actions if I plan to stay successful.

I decide to spend lunch break going over the notes I made on vascular disease last night in preparation for afternoon rounds. Before I can finish, I hear about a patient coming in from Jenkins, a small town about half an hour away. It is a Mr. Paul Bennett who was seen in the surgery outpatient clinic three weeks ago. Ben tells us that at that time, Mr. Bennett had a large abdominal aortic aneurysm along with some back pain. He reviewed the anatomy for us, explaining: "The aorta is the large artery that receives blood from the heart, traverses the chest and abdomen, and finally divides into the large arteries that go to the legs. Mr. Bennett's aorta is ballooning out in his abdomen, much like an inner tube will balloon out through a crack in a tire. This is called an aneurysm. An inner tube can rupture going 90 miles an hour on the highway or sitting still in the driveway. Similarly, it cannot be predicted when the aneurysm is going to rupture, so these aneurysms are usually taken out and replaced with a cloth tube as soon as they are discovered. If they manifest themselves by causing some pain in the back, as in Mr. Bennett's case, there is usually little time before it ruptures. I had seen Mr. Bennett in the clinic and had explained the seriousness of his aneurysm, but he had elected to wait a while on the operation. Ben begins to shake his head. "He has waited too long, because the aneurysm is now rupturing and he is on the way for a very bloody operation; his chances of survival are ten times worse now that he is leaking."

Within a few minutes, he is on the operating table with type specific blood being pumped into him. Mr. Bennett is breathing heavily and groaning with each breath. Both flanks are blue due to the blood leaking from the aneurysm. His feet have a waxy white appearance because no blood is reaching them. The look on his face is one of sheer terror. His eyes keep searching, but never finding. He looks anxiously at Ben, at me, at the I.V. pole, then his face relaxes as the sodium pentothal is injected and the merciful anesthetic begins to take its hold.

The chairman of surgery, Dr. Self, is present to assist on the operation. Ben quickly opens the abdomen from "tip to stern" and as soon as he enters the peritoneal cavity that holds all the intestines and abdominal organs, a huge blood clot can be seen around the aneurysm. "Get proximal control first," snaps Dr. Self.

Ben eases his hand up the aorta very slowly and deliberately to just above the beginning of the aneurysm. "I think it's above the kidney arteries," he says with a single negative movement of his head.

"Well, clamp it and let's go!" Dr. Self replies, underlining the necessity of speed in controlling the situation. From the reading I did last night, I know it is a bad prognostic sign if the aneurysm extends above where the arteries to the kidneys come off the aorta, as Ben is implying in this case. I also know that the survival rate of taking out a *ruptured* aneurysm and replacing it with a cloth graft is very low indeed. As Ben attempts to get control of the pulsating aorta, the bleeding begins. It looks like the dam broke. So much blood is coming out of the aorta, it literally fills up the peritoneal cavity. Ben finally gets the clamp placed across the vessel and the bleeding slows, but doesn't stop.

"Are you sure you have the whole thing clamped?" yells Dr. Self.

"I think so, but I don't have any idea where the arteries to the kidneys are located; don't want to clamp them," Ben replies.

"Go ahead and clamp the iliac arteries to the legs, and get it out of there," Dr. Self orders as he continues to suction blood out of the abdomen. There is still a considerable "ooze" even with the aorta clamped above and below the aneurysm, but Ben ignores this uncontrollable bleeding and steadily works at getting the aneurysm out.

The anesthesiologist at the head of the table pumps blood into the patient. "I don't get any blood pressure at all, and I am pumping in the twelfth unit now."

It seems a hopeless case, but Ben keeps sewing as fast as he can. The graft is in place; the clamps are removed—four hours have passed. The kidneys have not made any urine, there is still no blood pressure, he has been given eighteen units of blood, and is still bleeding from everywhere. Everything Ben touches bleeds. What else is there to do? The graft looks all right. There are no gross bleeding areas in the graft or where the graft is sewn to the aorta, but the blood continues to come from everywhere and all efforts at getting it stopped seem futile.

Dr. Self steps back from the table, takes off his gown and gloves and says, "Close him up. I'll go inform the family that things are going poorly."

Ben puts the last stitches in the abdomen. Blood fills the peritoneal cavity and seeps through the wound. Mr. Bennett is dying and Ben knows it, but he continues to work as hard as he can and gets him off the operating table and into the recovery room. I can't understand why all the details and rush. What difference does it make if he dies on the operating table or in the recovery room? He's going to die. I realize Ben has taken the whole responsibility for the patient. I am only a shadow of insignificance concerning Mr. Bennett, but I ask Ben some questions concerning my unsureness of the situation. He attempts to explain the recent action. "Have you ever played in a game where your team is way behind and you know you have no chance of winning? Well, whatever it is that makes you play those last two minutes as hard as you can is the same drive that makes me not want to have my patient expire on the operating table. Whether that 'something' is pride, hurt, care, concern, or hope for a miracle that the patient quits bleeding, I don't know."

Ben and I both know everything possible has been done, but we also know that his best was not enough to save the patient. Twenty minutes later, Mr Bennett dies in the recovery room.

Two weeks pass and Ben has yet to ask me to discuss vascular disease on rounds. Whether Mr. Bennett's death has anything to do with my not presenting, I'll never know. I also notice we have not had any more teaching sessions on vascular surgery. It appears to me that Ben has undergone an emotional setback because of the death of Mr. Bennett. It is difficult to understand why the death of this man would affect someone as self-assured as Ben appears. Perhaps I will know firsthand when I mature out of my cocoon of general surgery student into a full-bloomed chief resident. Evidently, there is more to surgery than operations.

Two days later, I meet Jack Sterns, a fellow classmate rotating on surgery with me. He is on the way to the operating room and complaining about having to scrub in on an open-heart operation. Such operations usually last most of the day, and students are not required to scrub and stand at the operating table for that length of time, but for some reason a request came out of the operating room that a student was wanted, and it happened to be Jack's patient.

"You really don't want to scrub on an open-heart operation?" I cannot believe he is not interested. I would give anything to actually be able to stand directly at the operating table of an open-heart.

"I have plenty of things I need to do other than stand and look at a heart all day." Jack continues to walk briskly down the hall toward the operating room, giving me only half his attention as I walk two steps behind.

"I'll scrub for you."

He stops so suddenly, I almost run into him.

"Are you kidding me?"

"No. I'll scrub. They don't know which student the patient belongs to anyway."

"Go to it. I think you're crazy, but go to it. I'll see you on evening rounds—you won't be out before then." Jack waves me on, and I continue the trek to the operating room.

It is exciting. I don't understand what is going on at the operating table, but at least I am getting a firsthand look at the apex of the surgical ladder, an open-heart operation. Afterwards, one of the students in our group tells me how lucky I was to get to scrub on an open-heart case. It all lies in the attitude as to whether my experience was a rose or a thorn. Positive attitude—a rose, negative attitude—a thorn. The operation was the same.

Once home with food in my stomach, I sit in the only stuffed chair in the house and recollect the day. I have learned the beginning of a lesson, I think. I was told I was "lucky" getting to scrub on the case. What really is luck? I have been told before that I was lucky in various happenings. All along the way, I believe I have been lucky in lots of ways. But I wonder. Today was not luck. I worked to be accepted to medical school. I worked to be on the surgical service. I worked to be in the position I was in today. And then the door of opportunity cracked open and let me see a glimpse of what was through the door—open-heart surgery. I walked on through the door and scrubbed on the case. Perhaps there is no such thing as luck. Perhaps all my previous luck is really just work, plus opportunity, plus action. Perhaps "how lucky you can get" is really "how hard have you prepared yourself to get into a position to act when an opportunity arrives." Perhaps, I don't know. I will put it to the test and see. Right now, I need to put myself to the test and get to reading surgery, or I will be unlucky tomorrow when questions start to be asked. I take enough time to write in my goal's book: Work plus opportunity plus action equals luck.

The next few days are spent mainly thinking about my becoming a surgeon. I get more excited the more I think of it. If I am to be a surgeon, now is the time to set the proper goals necessary to fulfill such a position. I will try to formulate these in my mind as I begin dog surgery. This portion of the rotation is spent actually performing operations on dogs. I will be able to act on my own ideas at an actual operating table in a true surgical setting. My immediate goal changes once again. I must take action to be the best dog surgeon I can possibly be. My attitude must be kept positive toward all the negative situations which will occur.

For dog surgery, we are divided into groups of four, with one student acting as the first surgeon, one the assistant, one the anesthesiologist, and one the scrub nurse to pass instruments. Before each operation, a real surgeon from the staff performs the procedure while we take notes on the technique of the operation and then perform it ourselves. There are four different operations planned, and each of us will be the first surgeon on one operation. As first surgeon I will actually get to do the cutting, as assistant I will act as the surgeon's helper; cut his knots, clamp bleeding arteries, retract tissue out of the way so he can see better, and do anything else he instructs me to do. There is much preparation. There are pages and pages to read about the associated disease and the surgery we will be doing and, in addition, we have to read all we can about how to put a dog to sleep and keep him alive during the procedure.

Dr. Wright is in charge of our dog surgery, and greets us with a stern face as we enter the dog lab for our first demonstration. The room is cold and bleak with no chairs, only the trough-like tables that hold the dogs. Dr. Wright is in his early fifties, has graying hair cut short, and is dressed in a green scrub suit covered by a long white lab coat. He neither smiles nor says any unnecessary words. As we gather around him, eager to hear every word, Dr. Wright discusses the operating tables. The setting is similar to our first day in anatomy, but now there is so much more excitement since we will be dissecting on live animals rather than cadavers.

"In the middle of the trough you will see this long thin pan which catches blood or irrigating solutions used during the operation. The pan drains into that bucket at the end of the table. The height of blood in your bucket tells how well you control bleeding during the operation. It can be a 'full bucket' case, a 'half bucket operation,' or a 'just covered the bottom' procedure. It's all a matter of pride—if you have any. I can teach a monkey to do these operations and I'll try to teach you. Anyone off the street can learn to operate, but only a surgeon knows when and why. I expect you to read all the assignments and have a thorough knowledge of the disease process related to the operation you are performing and be able to apply that to back up any decisions you make."

We seat ourselves on the floor in front of him as he hands out a list of references for each procedure. "You're expected to read and know the information covered in these references and any additional reading is up to you."

Just looking at the list I can't see how it is going to be physically possible to take enough time from our regular surgery rotation to read this additional material, much less read it well enough to be questioned.

"The first two procedures will be a splenectomy (removing the spleen) and a gastroenterostomy. All a gastroenterostomy entails is a communication made between the stomach and a piece of small intestine by cutting a hole in the side of the stomach, and another hole in the side of the intestine and sewing the two holes together so that food entering the stomach will fall through the hole into the intestine.

"There will be an oral exam following these first two procedures, after which you will perform a cholecystectomy (removing the gall bladder) and a small bowel resection. You will take out a portion of the small intestine and sew the two remaining ends together. That covers the operations, but does not cover everything you will be held responsible for. Anesthesia is vital to general surgery and not something to be taken for granted," he continues as he paces back and forth in front of our group. He seems to be in his own little world, talking and walking, looking at the floor, an occasional glance toward us. I am certain he must attain some satisfaction in flunking a student in dog surgery. This must be the most fun part of surgery rotation, but after listening to him, I think it may be the most difficult portion. "Anesthesia is vital to surgery, so we have made a rule. If any dog dies while under anesthesia, the one putting him to sleep has to write a paper on 'anesthesia deaths' with an adequate review of the literature."

Everyone begins to have a similar thought process. The deeper the dog is asleep, the greater the chance of an anesthetic death. As in the groups before us, each of us decides that when our turn comes to be anesthetist, the dog will be asleep just deeply enough to keep him on the table. After all, a live dog is better than a dead one, especially when a dead one means hours and hours of reviewing the literature and writing a paper.

Dr. Wright calls us to the scrub sink and starts his spiel on how to wash our hands prior to surgery: "The scrub consists of washing the hands and forearms initially just the way you do it at home before dinner. Next, take a scrub brush out of the sterile container and start scrubbing each finger, hand, and forearm for ten minutes. You will miss areas; to prove it, I'm going to have you do the 'black scrub.' I want you to paint this black dye on your hands and arms. I will blindfold you, let you scrub for ten minutes and then see what you have missed. If you scrub properly, the dye will come off—all of it." He points to a large plastic jar with the words "Black Scrub" painted on the side.

After applying the dye to our hands and arms, we scrub every inch of skin from elbows to finger tips for ten minutes. I feel sure I have covered the entire area more than adequately, and will surely be one of the few who ends up with no dye remaining on the skin. I remove my blindfold. There is black dye under my fingernails, the web of skin between each finger, and a whole strip up the back of each arm.

Dr. Wright picks up a scrub brush and starts a demonstration of the proper technique of scrubbing. "Scrub your fingertips and each web of skin between your fingers twenty times. Visualizing each finger as a four-sided box, scrub each side twenty times. Then scrub twenty times the back of each hand, your palms, and—again imagining a box—each side of your forearms. Then repeat the entire procedure, this time scrubbing each area only ten times." Dr. Wright briskly goes through the scrub for us and begins to rinse off the soap. "When rinsing, hold your hands up and your elbows down, so that the water always runs from the tips of your fingers, a cleaned area, toward your elbows, which is considered a contaminated area. In this way, dirty water from around your elbows will not run back down onto the areas just scrubbed."

The first day in dog surgery ends with all of us back at the scrub sink trying to get the black dye washed from under our fingernails.

I stop by the operating room of the hospital on the way home and ask one of the nurses for some silk suture to practice tying knots. "This ought to do you," she says as she gives me a handful of 2-0 silk suture. "We'll give you more when you are ready for one hand knots," she laughs.

I know there are two ways to tie knots, a two handed tie which is similar to tying shoelaces with both hands, and a one handed knot which is much quicker, but more difficult to learn. I will stick to learning the two handed method for now.

After supper, I set my chair directly in front of the refrigerator while Harriet does the dishes. I clumsily begin practicing tying knots on the door handle. One hour later I announce: "Okay, time me." Harriet plays my game and tells me when to begin. One minute later I have tied forty-four knots. I mentally set a goal of one hundred before I finish my surgery rotation.

Three nights later I decide to try one hand knots. They can be tied much more rapidly than the two hand knots once you learn them, but I only do eight in the first minute. My fingers just don't "think" that way. I glance at the refrigerator door handle on the way to bed; hundreds of black silk sutures dangle loosely. Those silk sutures represent more than the fact that my fingers are ready for surgery. It has become a symbol in my mind. Tied silk sutures on the refrigerator door handle are some tangible representation of my major goal: to become a surgeon. The actual thread would be worth perhaps fifty cents to the average citizen. But, to me, it is worth hours and hours of study, and numerous immediate actions performed. I suppose symbols have always been important to me. Just as these silk surgical threads tell me I am a surgeon, the ball point pen advertising a drug company tells me I am a medical student, and buying a small wooden box filled with dissecting instruments for frog anatomy told me I was a pre-medical student. All of the symbols are worth very little to anyone other than an aspiring surgeon, medical student, or a pre-medical college student. But for me, it is a strong reinforcement for the goal set in my mind. And for some reason, which perhaps a psychiatrist can tell me, I want to leave those silk sutures on the refrigerator door handle. They are my trophies and encouragement. They reinforce the fact that I will become a surgeon. In my mind, they represent that I am now a surgeon and that is the way I see myself tonight. Because I know I will achieve my goal, I can see myself as already having achieved it. I look back at the definition of success written only a few days ago in the *Goal's Rule Book*: I am successful as long as I am working toward my major goal.

I go to bed feeling very successful and ready for our first day of "live" dog surgery. As I lie in bed, I think back over the black scrub routine a few days ago. The word "honesty" comes to mind. How honest am I with myself? Do I apply a "black scrub policy" to the way I look at things that really matter? I know in some instances, I put on a blindfold and say something, or do something, that can probably get me by just the way it is. But what about taking the blindfold off and really seeing what it is that I am saying or doing? Would things stand up to Dr. Wright's black scrub policy of acknowledging, that after all, I am not "one of the few" to whom the policy does not apply.

Our dog surgery team consists of the original "Minnie group." For the first case Charles Wilson is first surgeon, I am assistant, Bill Warren is anesthesiologist, and Pokie is the surgical nurse. Of all people to put the dog to sleep on our first case, Bill is the worst possible selection.

"It's going to be hard, Charlie. Bill's going to keep the dog light, as scared as he is of the dog dying on him." I almost whisper to Charlie as we scrub for the case while Bill makes ready to put the dog to sleep.

"It will be hard enough for me to get the gall bladder out if the dog were dead, much less moving all over the table." Charlie says, closing his eyes and shaking his head.

Time to start! We scrub the dog's abdomen, drape him out, and Charlie gets knife in hand. "The dog is not asleep yet," Bill says gruffly. "I'll let you know when to cut." Bill is busy trying to get the dog into the correct depth of anesthesia by dropping ether onto a mask covering the dog's nose and mouth. So we stand, waiting for Bill to get the dog to sleep enough to operate on. After ten minutes Bill says we can start and Charlie puts the knife on the abdomen and barely makes a nick. The dog almost jumps off the table. We both respond quickly in order to hold the sterile sheet in place. Bill mumbles a few words and hastens to get more ether into the mask. There is so much commotion that everybody in the room looks over at our table.

"That's real good, Bill," one of our classmates yells.

"No chance of his dying of anesthesia," quips another, "You haven't used enough ether to put a gnat to sleep." Everyone is laughing by this time. Everyone except us. Bill's face is so red I don't know whether he is embarrassed, or getting ready to explode. After a time we proceed, the remainder of the operation proving to be a struggle, mainly because the dog is not in deep sleep, and partly because this is our first case. The procedure completed, our group of four makes a mutual decision; from now on the surgeon will tell the anesthesiologist how much asleep he wants the dog while the operation is going on, and if the dog dies, we will all pitch in and help write the paper on "death under anesthesia." At least, if we all work toward the same goal of helping the surgeon, we will all come out ahead.

Sure enough, once we begin to work together with the same goal in mind, the operations become easier and faster. All we needed was a oneness; something to make us work together. That oneness was agreed upon by all to help the one acting as surgeon of the day.

This is a good point. Looking back it is easy to see now that when each of us worked as separate individuals, there was nothing but chaos. One centered only on putting the dog to sleep, another only on the operation, another on how neat to keep the instruments, and the other tried to assist the surgeon. But once we put our minds together and decided to all work toward the one goal of helping the one doing the operation, everything worked much better. The one acting as scrub nurse became interested in what was going on at the operating table rather than just trying to keep the instruments wiped clean. If help was needed at a difficult point in the procedure, he would lend a hand. The assistant to the surgeon became more interested in what was going on and became a second surgeon on the case rather than just an assistant who had to be told everything to be done. Even the anesthesiologist paid more attention to keeping the dog asleep and relaxed, especially when we encountered a difficult part of the operation.

In fact, it was almost like having an extra hand at the operating table. This has proved to be a real phenomena. Once our gang decided on the same goal of making the operation go as well as possible, then, and only then, did we acquire the extra hand phenomena.

We end up giving the dogs more care and attention than any of the patients we are following in the hospital. I do not want the dogs I operate on to die in post-op. I am sure a good portion of this feeling is for my ego rather than for the benefit of the dog. Nevertheless, I personally feed the dog I operated on twice a day. As we complete the section of surgery rotation to be done at the university hospital, dog surgery comes to an end. Eight operations in our newly named "Goal Group": no deaths, no massive hemorrhage, and no major complications—and no anesthesia paper to write!

Later that night at home, Harriet and I both finish our book work early. For the past several days I have been reflecting on the smoothness with which dog surgery went after we all decided to work together toward one goal. I think this same principle should work in marriage as well, so I decide to put it to the test.

I put my feet up on the stool and move to one side of the overstuffed chair—my favorite study spot. Then, motioning for Harriet to sit beside me, I say, "Come on over." She squeezes in sideways and snuggles up to me as I place my right arm around her shoulders and give her a squeeze.

"I've been thinking about our money situation." I speak to her, but I put my head on the back of the chair and look straight ahead.

"We're not doing badly, are we?" She looks up at me questioningly.

"No, but we don't have a plan. We save a little, spend a little, and give some to the church. Let's set a goal. Let's give ten percent to the church and put ten percent in savings. We can do it."

"You have to cut out Cokes at lunch. We can't do it and buy Cokes."

"How about making me a lunch everyday, a couple of sandwiches or so?" I respond, happy that Harriet has accepted the idea of setting this goal. I am realizing something that is becoming more and more apparent as our marriage progresses. It is important for both of us to develop the same goals and work toward them together. That makes for a greater sense of oneness.

So, as we begin working on our saving and giving program, I begin the last portion of the surgery rotation, which is at the Veteran's Administration hospital. It has been converted from an old resort hotel into a hospital, the grounds kept as they were in the 1930's with huge trees scattered around the front lawn and five acres of lush green grass. The hospital itself is a four-story, white painted brick building. The old golf course is still preserved in excellent condition behind the hospital. There is definitely a sense of relaxation and informality here in contrast to the university hospital I just left. It even seems more appropriate to be carrying a lunch here, than at the university hospital.

I am the first student to arrive on this initial day of the V.A. rotation. There is one resident in the surgery office flipping through the latest issue of one of the monthly issues of *Annals of Surgery* while leaning back in his chair, feet propped up on the table.

"Come on in. My name is Charlie Stern. Call me Charlie. Make yourself at home, coffee's in the bathroom. The rest of the crew will be here shortly." Charlie is a tall lanky man about thirty years old, wears his black hair longer than usual; keeps most of it brushed out of his face. He puts the surgery journal down. "I'm a third year resident. Bruce Conner is first year, and John Baker is chief. We don't have any interns out here. John runs a loose service, lets us do pretty much as we like. You play golf?"

Less than sixty seconds have passed, and I already know Charlie. I have heard a lot about him from other students. He is known as the student's friend, doesn't mind taking up time teaching and talking with students, and is supposed to be very practical in patient care and lets the students do as much "cutting" as possible. This usually amounts to taking off moles and lipomas—fatty tumors.

The other students arrive, and Charlie orients us to the floors and office. John Baker, the chief resident, comes in only long enough to announce that he is going out of town. He glances at Charlie, "Take them on rounds and see if you can't get Pollard's temperature down today. He might have an abscess."

How different it is out here from the university hospital. There, we had a routine for everything, and a time and place for everything. Here, the residents work whenever they want so long as the work gets done.

John turns toward our student group and continues with his instructions: "We don't have any surgery scheduled this morning, so split up the patients and write an up-to-date 'on-service note' on the chart giving the summary of the patient's history and course while in the hospital. This will be beneficial for a quick reference review when you have to present your patient on rounds or in a conference." John leaves following his short appearance for the day.

"You come with me," Charlie says pointing to me. "Understand you're interested in going into surgery."

I am not sure how he knows that fact, but evidently he has taken enough initiative to research the students coming on his service. No one has ever mentioned my going into surgery directly to me, and I feel awkward discussing my future following such a superficial acquaintance. I hesitate and then reply.

"I hope to, if the time ever comes for me to finish med school."

"I'm in charge of assigning new patients to the students. You just take all my patients and work them up when they come in and then you work with me. When I come in early, you be here; when I have to stay late, you stay late. Now, I occasionally sleep late when I don't have an early case. I'll let you know the day before and you can do the same. Oh yes, I play golf every Thursday afternoon. Students are scheduled for a conference with Dr. Dover at that time, but you skip and I'll teach you a few new swings with the clubs. Old Dover is a terrible teacher and everybody ends up falling asleep before it's over anyway. You won't miss a thing."

I fit into the pattern Charlie sets up and find I have a little more work to do than normally expected on the V.A. rotation, but it is well worth it. By the third week, I have scrubbed on a total of fourteen hernias and am sure I can do one. I decide to discuss the situation with Charlie to see if there is any possibility of such an event.

I catch him in his office. "You know, Mr. Barker, the hernia that came in today? It certainly does feel like a small one."

Charlie puts down the journal he is reading and smiles. "Buba," (the name he calls all the students) "I guess you're gonna tell me it's so small that even Bruce won't want to do it."

I sit down, but say nothing.

"All right, if it is okay with Bruce, I'll let you steal it from him."

Those are the very words I wanted to hear. "It's fine with Bruce; I've already asked him," I reply.

"You fox you, I'll tell you what. I'll let you start the case and go as far as you can. When you start bogging down, Bruce takes over. Fair enough?" Charlie becomes serious in his manner.

"You give me an hour and a half to finish and I'll guarantee you I'll get it done correctly." I really feel good. This is an unusual opportunity for me because there is no intern on the service, and Bruce has done more hernias than he wants and doesn't mind turning the case over to Charlie and me.

Fifty-two minutes and I did it all. I even surprise myself with how fast the operation goes. It marks the high point of my career to this date. I go to the doctors' dressing room to change out of my scrub suit. I have just performed an actual operation! Elation is no word to describe my feelings. I could not be more satisfied than any surgeon who has just completed his first open-heart surgery case. I have been given a small nibble of what it is all about, and I hunger for more.

I realize desire has just been given a boost. What makes desire build in a person? What causes the hunger to reach the proportions that make me want to do a hernia operation? And now, it is even greater. It is a *compelling desire* that centers all thoughts around one goal—that of becoming a surgeon. That is the direct offspring of that small, *initial desire* to become a surgeon; the desire I had after finishing high school! I know that this compelling desire is related to that original desire. And now that I have actually performed an operation, the original desire has been rekindled tenfold. I am glad I acted on the initial desire in high school. Looking back, the initial desire seems so small and insignificant. It is like a fetus still in the uterus compared with the compelling desire I now have. There is no doubt in my mind that I would have made all "As" in college if my "fetal" desire had matured into a compelling desire before I started college. I must keep this in mind the next time I have a small inkling to do something. I must look ahead and see what the outcome might be if that desire matured into a compelling desire. I bet it would multiply my potential tenfold in whatever I undertook.

Right now, I had better come down off my cloud and think about how much of a surgeon I really am. Charlie lets me write the admitting orders on the chart; he lets me write the post-op orders after surgery; he has even let me perform an operation. But, I really do not have day control over the patient. If my orders are incorrect, he changes them; if I had started to make one wrong move at the operating table, he would have taken over. He, not I, is in charge of the patient's well-being. None of my decisions is worth writing in the chart without Charlie's approval. True, I can learn from these experiences, but I must never let the little corner of my mind labeled "make-believe doctor" grow to include any of my useful mind. I must reserve the useful portion for reality. It is real; I am still just a medical student with ninety-nine pages out of a hundred yet to learn.

I do not get to do any more major surgery during my stay at the V.A., but I do pick up some of the basic knowledge I need to become an M.D. and finish the rotation with a self-satisfaction I have never before experienced. I have taken the first real steps toward becoming a surgeon and regret that the over-all rotation is nearing an end. I have also kindled the desire to become a surgeon to the point that it is now a compelling hunger, a compelling desire.

As the surgery rotation ends, I leave with a generally satisfying memory of what I have just gone through. I have matured quickly having to face the realities of life and death. Not all patients get well; not all patients just have a baby and go home. Some have an incurable cancer and no matter how much surgery is performed, no matter how much medicine is given, no matter how "good" a patient is, that particular patient is going to die. This is difficult for me to accept, but I have been exposed.

It has been a good rotation, one I hate to leave. But there is much more general medicine yet to be learned and so I start the last rotation of my junior year in medical school: internal medicine. It is a speciality that deals with diagnosing a disease and treating it with medicine. There are many overlaps between medical and surgical patients, and these two divisions of medicine must work together in giving the individual patient the best possible care. Patients with diabetes, heart failure, chronic kidney disease, lung problems, hematological diseases, and many chronic multiple systems diseases frequently develop coexisting surgical problems which necessitate operations regardless of the associated medical difficulties. In such cases, it is important for the surgeon to realize the severity of the medical problem and seek advice from his medical associates. It is equally important for the internist with patients who have a surgically related disease to consult the surgeon early. However, as with much overlapping situations in life, certain surgeons and internists have little regard for each other's ability to care for the patient, thus the old adage: "An internist knows everything, but does nothing" (according to surgeons). "A surgeon knows nothing, but does everything" (according to internists).

Since I know I am going into surgery, I start medicine rotation with less enthusiasm than I had at the beginning of the surgery rotation. I can find interest in medical problems that are in some way related to surgery, but find it very difficult to force myself to read about diseases I will never see nor treat, having to constantly remind myself I should do the best I can if for no other reason than grades—all important in being accepted to a good internship program.

I think back to my college days where no course in particular seemed to be of significance in actually helping me to some day become a doctor. Yet, each course was necessary for me to graduate from college and be acceptable for medical school. I can fit this situation of studying medicine, when I would rather be studying surgery, into that same category. This has become a similar situation to a year ago when I needed to study. I must make my immediate actions goal to learn all I can about internal medicine in order to finish medical school and be accepted to a surgical program. In this way, I can look over and beyond the immediate difficulties and keep my eyes focused on the intermediate goal of completing medical school. I look at this as GOAL REASONING rather than tricking my mind. I reason one step ahead, keeping the major goal always in the back of my mind. Goal reasoning is being able to look beyond the immediate actions at hand and seeing the final accomplishment of the intermediate and major goals completed.

Once again I feel this is worth writing in the book because it has helped me before and will help me now.

GOAL REASONING: The ability to look beyond, the ability to see the major goal accomplished in order to cope with the present situation. With this in mind, I return my actions and thought to internal medicine. We are required to work up three patients a week, doing a complete physical examination, making a diagnosis, reading literature concerning the particular disease, and then writing a long summation concerning the particular patient.

"I want you to learn how to work up a patient correctly," states Dr. Franks, the chief of the medicine service. An aging man of sixty-five, he has a hatchet face with little expression other than a forced smile now and then. His beady, dark eyes are accented by his habit of staring at a single student while talking. Whether this staring has any significance depends entirely upon the conscience of the student at whom he is looking. Dr. Franks is nearing retirement age, but is not slowing in his interest to teach students. He expects a certain amount of work from us, and receives it—either from respect by the student, or by humiliation from Dr. Franks. I take notes as he begins a lecture he has given thousands of students before.

"I don't want any two-page work-ups like you did on surgery. I want ten pages and I want you to write down all the negative findings as well as the positive. That's the only way you're ever going to remember to ask the patient all the questions you need in a complete examination. I also want correct spelling and I want to be able to read your writing—even if you have to print. You can get away with sloppy writing on the other services, but not on mine. There is a specific way I want patients worked up and that is the way it will be done on this service. When you get on pediatrics, O.B., or surgery, you can work them up any way you want, but here you'll do it the way I tell you because I think this is the best way to learn to cover all aspects of the patient as well as the specific disease the patient has." Dr. Franks walks over to the blackboard and writes "C.C."

"You begin with the 'chief complaint' of the patient. This should be a few words stating what the patient is complaining of and should be written in the patient's own words."

"P.I." is written just under "C.C." on the board.

"Next comes 'present illness,' and this should include a narrative summary of the patient's illness, when he first began to complain of his symptoms, what brought the symptoms on, how long they lasted, and if there was anything which relieved them. This is to be in detail and should cover all aspects of the illness. Pain has many different meanings to different individuals, and you have to decide the significance of the pain the patient is describing as related to his illness. Some patients will be very sick and express little pain, while others may express a lot of pain with only minor irritations." Dr. Franks has everyone's attention. Each student is busy taking notes on how the professor wants his patients written up; no one wants to miss a single instruction because we know the work will have to be redone if it does not meet with his approval.

He writes "P.H." on the board and continues his lecturing.

"The 'past history' should include the patient's occupation, habits concerning smoking and drinking, unusual childhood diseases, adult diseases, family history, operations, injuries and allergies. If you don't ask the patient these questions, you may miss something important to the over-all treatment."

"R.O.S." is the fourth line written on the board.

"A 'review of systems' is a review of every system of the body, and I want each system investigated in detail on every patient and a statement made for each system. You will start with the general physical condition of the patient and then start with the head and work down. Ask the patient if he has ever had any diseases or injuries related to the head, eyes, ears, nose, or throat. I want each of these listed separately; you will not use statements as 'within normal limits,' 'negative,' or 'not remarkable.' If you ask the patient ten questions about his ears and all the answers are normal, then write down each question and state that the patient is healthy in each aspect. Neck: ask for any history of lumps, pain or injuries related to the neck. Next, discuss lung problems; any history of pneumonia, spitting up blood, chronic cough, T.B. or infections. Ask the patient questions. If you don't, you're going to miss something, and I will know if you leave anything out on my patient.

"The cardiovascular system is next and this is to include any form of heart disease or peripheral vascular disease. You may pick up early heart failure just by asking the right questions. Ask if his ankles swell at the end of the day. He may be unaware of the swelling. Ask him if his shoes feel tighter in the evening than in the morning. That may be the only clue you get that he is having mild congestive heart failure. We can treat that, you know."

On and on he goes. I already have written over two pages of instructions of just questions to ask the patient and he is not through yet. I can see that medicine work-ups will take as much time to write as an entire operation took on surgery.

"You can ask a hundred questions on this next system and still not cover it adequately—the G.I. tract. This includes anything to do with the esophagus, stomach, small intestines, colon, and rectum. Cover it all: ulcers, diarrhea, bleeding, hemorrhoids, and consistency of the stool. Some of these diseases we can treat and some we have to give to the surgeons. Don't ever send a patient you haven't worked up completely to a surgeon. If you do, and he finds something on the patient you missed, it's an unforgivable sin . . . unforgivable. I will admit, if you just look at a patient from ten yards away, you will learn more about him than any surgeon who spends an hour examining him, but there is the outside chance he will stumble onto something." He smiles gently with the statement, that being the first sign the old man has any humor at all. He even turns the corners of his mouth up slightly as he continues, "You know the old saying. . . .'Even a blind hog will find an acorn now and then by chance.'"

Everyone laughs, taking this as an opportunity to stretch our fingers and hoping the laughter might delay the lecture a few moments. I am getting writer's cramp trying to keep up with the "outline" Dr. Franks is giving.

For the next thirty minutes, he discusses the genito-urinary, gynecological, lymphatic, musculo-skeletal, and neuro-psychiatric systems.

"And last, and almost least, comes the physical examination. Do you know what percentage of pertinent information you can get from the physical alone? Ten percent. If a patient walks into your office and you do nothing but a physical examination, you would have only ten percent of the information you need to treat him. That's why I want you to spend ninety percent of your time talking with the patient before you ever start the examination."

Dr. Franks pauses. He stares at the only female student in our group. "I'm sure you all know how to do a physical examination; they can at least teach you that much in surgery." Through the years, he has developed a fondness for making jabs at the surgeons—the other side of the coin. "Cover everything we covered on review of systems and write down your findings. In the past there have been two parts of the examination that the students seem to get into the habit of leaving out—the pelvic exam on females and the rectal exam on males. I want these exams done on each patient by the resident, intern, and student. You cannot learn it by reading what someone else found on their examinations. I also don't want to have three exams at separate times. You get with the resident and intern and do this part of the exam at the same meeting." Dr. Franks places his piece of chalk on the table and leaves the room. There is silence for a few seconds, and then noise mounts as everyone begins to complain about the length of the work-ups.

Looking over the outline, I see why we only work up three patients a week. It will take all day to write up a patient the way he wants: But if that is the way he wants it, that is the way I will do it. It is going to be a long three months; I would rather be operating than writing up patients. I need this rotation, however, and know it is essential in rounding out my medical education. I once again remind myself of *goal reasoning: look beyond.* My *immediate action* goal is to do the best I can on the medicine rotation. *Immediate action goals* call for action—right now! I will have to remind myself of this a thousand times the next three months and apply all the goal reasoning I can muster to get through all this paper work.

There are so many diversified diseases treated on the medical service that I soon build respect for the difficult cases. Diabetes, heart conditions, leukemia, renal failure—all of these have to be treated by specialists in each field. Vast knowledge has to be learned and applied with trials of different medications to successfully treat these patients. After two months on Medicine, I have settled into a routine of almost a nine-to-five job except for the long nightly reading sessions required to keep up on this service.

Harriet and I have come to like our small three-room garage apartment and especially the nicety of the tin roof. On this particular night, as usual, she has gone to bed, leaving me sitting by myself reading the textbook of Internal Medicine. It begins to rain. Nothing quite compares with the sound of a good hard rain starting off with only a little drop here and then another one there. But not being able to keep up with the changing positions of the sounds, I let the book drop into my lap as my head falls back to rest on the cushioning of the chair. I always reward myself with the pleasure of listening to it rain on the tin. My mind begins to wander: "What makes someone go into internal medicine? Why would anyone go into pediatrics and have to treat all those screaming babies? Who would want to go into O.B. and have to get up in the middle of the night to deliver a baby? That's when they always seem to be born. Why doesn't everybody go into surgery? Most of the patients are cured and back home a week after the operation. The patients are grateful because they came with something wrong and a few days later it has been taken care of. And above all, it is very satisfying to perform and accomplish something with your hands." These thoughts jog through my mind as I slouch further down into the chair and allow my eyelids to relax. "I'm glad not everyone wants to go into surgery . . . that would mean I might have to go into Internal Medicine and do those long work-ups the rest of my life . . ." I awake at four o'clock and realize I dozed for two hours. The sleep-enducing rain has stopped, but I have no trouble crawling into bed and dropping back off to sleep.

I begin in the portion of the medicine rotation which is spent at the city hospital. I keep noticing an elderly, wiry little gentleman in the men's ward, first bed on the right. He doesn't appear sick and always speaks each time I pass his bed. On inquiring as to the diagnosis of the patient and why he has been in the hospital so long, I am informed he has been in the same bed for over a year. Diagnosis? "Nothing specific."

I decide to stop and talk since I have a few minutes before the lecture begins. I introduce myself and soon am in a most intriguing conversation with an eighty-seven-year-old man without a single hair to cause his head to itch, yet he frequently rubs it; without a tooth in his mouth, yet he constantly shows his gums with a broad smile. He was a barber in his younger days—a "doctorin' barber then," as he puts it.

"I used to treat high blood pressure." He answers my ignorance of ancient barbers. "I cut the jugular vein, let it run down into a little curved basin that fit around their neck. Looked like a dinner plate with a piece taken out of one side. When the basin was full, I'd just hold pressure on the vein until it quit bleeding."

"Ever have one who wouldn't quit bleeding?" I ask, feeling that I have just stumbled into Alley Oop's time machine and found myself in ancient medicine.

"One," he answers honestly. I do not question him about it further.

I feel a certain satisfaction as I leave the old man in bed number one. I invested ten minutes of free time and received, as a dividend, a story out of the history book of medicine, told in first person. I treasure my ten minutes with him more than the hour lecture I am about to attend. I am sure I will remember his "lecture" years after I forget the formal medicine lecture of the day.

I continue my routine for another month and find that with the end of this rotation at hand and still so much reading to be done, it will be impossible to complete. I leave the service with neither the taste of honey nor lemon. I have not disliked it but neither have I the desire to pursue such studies. The one thing I do come away with is the realization that some internists and some surgeons disagree on treatment of some patients, and both let professional pride get in the way of deciding the proper, beneficial treatment of the patient. They don't mean to and only a few in each camp fall into this category. The goal group phenomena which I learned in dog surgery definitely should be applied to these cases. The best possible care of the patient should be placed as the goal, and the group of internists and surgeons should work together with that in mind. I have seen doctors work together as a goal group with the results being beautiful care for the patient. I have seen doctors work on the same patient, but as individuals independent of one another with much poorer results.

With the ending of the medicine rotation, the junior year of medical school is completed. There is a three-month break in the schedule between the junior and senior years, but not in actuality. This supposed "free time" period allows the hospital to hire students for special projects. Plus, this gives me the opportunity to get a job, make some much needed money to live on, as well as to travel around the country and apply for internship programs. Once the senior year begins, it will be difficult to get away to look at the different internship programs, so I will put this block of time to good use.

I apply and am accepted as an "extern" in the surgery department for the next three-month break. The job pays two hundred dollars a month, which is a welcome treat to supplement the income that Harriet makes in her teaching job. My new job consists of working with the surgery interns and residents; working up patients; operating with the interns and residents; and doing some of the post-operative care. It's almost like being an intern except I will not have the responsibility for the care of the patient and will consider it luck if any of the operations are passed down to me. Eight students are selected for the job, all of whom plan to go into surgery.

With the job problem taken care of, I look beyond my senior year and begin considering the different types of internships available. I can do a straight medicine internship, which would be twelve months of medicine with no surgery or pediatrics. Dr. Baxter, my student advisor, suggests I seriously consider doing such an internship since I will be doing surgery the rest of my life and will never again have the opportunity to study internal medicine for any length of time. This makes sense but it seems like a waste of a year I could be using in surgery.

A second choice is a "rotating" or "mixed" internship in which I can rotate among medicine, surgery, and pediatrics, spending four months on each service.

The final alternative is a straight surgery internship, spending the entire year in surgery. This is what I desire, but Dr. Baxter persists in recommending a straight medicine internship. He is a surgeon and he took a straight medicine internship; *he's not the best of surgeons, however.* Weighing each consideration through carefully, I decide on a mixed internship of medicine, surgery, and pediatrics even though I would rather spend the entire year in surgery.

This entails another major decision. Should I go to a "teaching" hospital where there is a full-time staff paid to do research and teach, or should I go to a private city hospital where I may get to do more surgery, make a lot more money as an intern, but not have the benefit of a full time teacher. There are good and bad points to both systems and many say it doesn't matter which program you enter because you get out of it what you put into it. Most of the teaching programs are available at state medical schools similar to this school. The non-teaching programs are offered at anything from small community hospitals to large county hospitals. I can make almost twice as much money in a non-teaching program and this fact alone is enticing after four years of financial struggle in medical school.

I look one year beyond internship in making my decision. I want to get a good surgery residency. The rest of my practicing years in surgery will be based on what I learn during residency, so I should probably try to get an internship in the same program at the same hospital. I will stand a better chance getting a good residency if I am already in the program as an intern. Therefore, I decide on a teaching hospital for internship.

I narrow my choice to four hospitals and fill out the long applications to each. I make plans to take off the last week in August for an interview at each hospital. Not only will I have to choose which hospital I want, but I will have to be lucky enough for that particular hospital to choose me. I sign up for the "matching plan" which means that on a certain date I will list the hospitals I have made application to in order of preference. On the same date each hospital across the country will hand in a list of students they are willing to accept as interns in order of preference. Both lists will be fed into a computer and if the hospital I pick chooses me, there is a "match" and I will do my internship there. If my first choice hospital does not pick me, then my name slips down to my second choice hospital to see if there is a match; and if not, on down the line my name goes until I match with a hospital that has listed my name on their preference list.

Harriet and I decide to make the week of interviews double as our vacation, and she will join me in my travels. We borrow her parents' car since our Volkswagen is pushing eighty thousand miles, and I surely don't want to miss such important appointments due to car trouble.

Harriet has adjusted well in the transition from a college student who is dependent on her parents for financial support, to chief breadwinner and wife of a husband who is rarely home. She keeps a neat apartment, is an excellent cook, and speaks frequently of having our first child. When I compare what she got when she married me, to what I got when I married her, I realize that I overmarried. I got a better deal than she.

We discuss how important these internship interviews are as we head toward our first destination. I am nervous about the interviews, but Harriet is very supportive and encouraging. I know that with her support everything will turn out all right.

I am interviewed at two university hospitals, both with great programs, however, neither has that something special to make me wholeheartedly want to go there. We head for the third interview, tired of traveling, tired of eating hamburgers, tired of pushing to get to the next appointment by a specific date, and most of all, I am tired of being interviewed.

In this frame of mind, we arrive at the third and final hospital on my list. It is a fairly new building since the medical school is only five years old; however, I have heard so many good reports about its surgery program I do not see how it can be so good and yet so young. We arrive late in the evening and pass the hospital for a look at the outside. What an impressive sight. There is a lighted fountain in front with a neatly kept lawn and shrubbery silhouetted against an array of floodlights. Over the entrance to the hospital is a huge marble mural of contrasting colored marble figures. The hospital looks great from the outside; if only the surgical program looks as great inside. I will have an opportunity to find out soon enough; my first interview is scheduled for eight o'clock in the morning.

Since I am applying for a "mixed internship," my first interview is with an internal medicine staff physician. He asks me where I am from, what I plan to go into after internship, and what my outside interests are. I mention working on a 1929 Model A Ford Roadster intermittently for the past several years, whenever I had time. This is about as far as we go in the interview because he is also interested in old cars, so we spend the remaining twenty-five minutes talking about antique automobiles.

That was an enjoyable discussion, but I don't see how he can arrive at any conclusions about my ability to be an intern by talking about Model A's. Bad interview, I think to myself as I look for the next office on my list. Dr. Peterson, pediatrics. Room H-202—nine A.M. I glance down the list of interviews and notice I am interviewed by an internist, a pediatrician and an orthopedic surgeon. No general surgeons on the list. General surgery is what I am most interested in and no interview.

The remaining interviews go as most—questions, answers, smiles, and small notes written by the interviewer. No one tries to sell me on coming to this hospital after I tell them I have decided on general surgery. The more I ask about the general surgery residency program the more it seems apparent that the head of general surgery is only interested in "straight surgery" interns. Dr. Don Eler is the chairman of the Department of Surgery and is nationally known to run a tight ship. The only conclusion I reach is that I have to get an interview with him if I am to have a chance of getting into his residency program. The entire morning has been a waste of time as far as I am concerned. If I am going to get into Dr. Eler's program, I must sell myself directly to him.

I drop by his office after finishing my last interview and ask his secretary if I can possibly have an appointment with him.

"You'll never get an appointment," she laughs. "He's in and out of here all day. You can take a seat and see if you can catch him for a minute between cases. He's too busy to be bothered by having to be here at a particular time, but he will always take time from his schedule if we can only catch him. I'll do all I can for you."

I sit down and begin going over in my mind exactly what I am going to say to Dr. Eler to convince him to accept me in his program.

An intern walks into the office.

"Is Dr. Eler around?"

"No, he's still in surgery and I have no idea when he'll be out," the secretary replies hardly looking up from her typing.

"I need to talk to him about a patient. Will you page me when he comes back to the office?"

"I will, but you know how he is. He will be gone again by the time you get down here. You had better try to catch him yourself."

As they talk, it occurs to me it would be a good idea to get this intern aside and get the real low-down on the internship program, as well as his opinion of Dr. Eler.

"Excuse me, I'm here looking at the internship program and wonder if I could talk with you a few moments?" The intern nods and motions me into the hall and on into the resident's office.

"Hey, I'm Charlie Johnson. What would you like to know?" Charles has the personality that makes me feel as if I had known him all my life. He is dressed in a gray scrub suit and cap, with a paper scrub mask hanging around his neck. He still has his operating shoes on which were green at one time, but now have so many blood stains, they have turned a dark brown everywhere except the heel portion. He has a natural smile and his ruffled, curly hair curls around his cap edges. He takes a seat and waits for me to speak.

"I am looking for an internship and at the same time a surgical residency. I figure to stand a better chance getting accepted in the residency program if I were around for a year as an intern. I like to operate and heard this was the place to come to do a lot of cutting."

Charles breaks in, "Well, you heard right. I came here from the University of Virginia as a mixed intern, but after two months on surgery I talked them into letting me switch to straight surgery. I've already done more hernias than you can shake a stick at and my resident is going to let me do a gall bladder next week. You know you aren't going to get to do that anywhere else—especially this early in the year."

"I know. You have to be a first or second year resident to get a gall bladder where I come from," I chime in.

"Most places are like that. The older schools pretty well have a tradition concerning which cases belong to the intern, which ones to the first year resident, and on up the line. If you don't get to do a gall bladder until you are a second year man, you sure aren't going to turn around and give it away to a man under you. That's what makes this place so nice. It's young enough that the chief resident is passing good cases down to the junior resident, and in turn he passes good cases down to the intern. You won't find another residency like it." Charles is very enthusiastic about the program and, at least in his mind, is sure there is none better. "The boss—that's what everybody calls Dr. Eler—really pushes you, too. He believes if you are capable of doing a certain operation, you should be allowed to do it, no matter what year of training you happen to be in. If you are good, you can advance fast, and if you are not good, he will probably kick you out of the program.

"Look, I've got to get back over to the operating room. If you have time stay awhile and make rounds with me this afternoon."

"When and where do you begin?"

"About six-thirty—seventh floor." With that, Charles smiles and heads back toward the O.R.

"This is the place I have been looking for," I think as I walk back into Dr. Eler's reception room. "I've just got to get an internship here. If they will have me, I'm not looking any further." I become more and more anxious as I wait. "What if he's too busy to see me?" I don't feel like my interviews here were that good; nothing went wrong, but they weren't that good either. I'll have to see Dr. Eler even if it means staying over and coming back tomorrow. With no one to talk to, my mind has nothing to do but convince me of it's decision.

Twelve o'clock. One o'clock. Two o'clock. At two-fifteen a tall, lean surgeon in scrub clothes with a long white coat flapping behind bursts through the door, hurries through the reception room and into his office. His door slams shut.

He didn't even see me. I hope he didn't see me; if he did, I don't think he wants to talk to me, slamming the door like that.

I am not sure what to say to the secretary.

"He probably didn't even see you. Let me call him on the intercom." She pushes the red button on her phone and I hear a buzzer sound in his office.

"There is a doctor here . . . concerning an internship. He has been waiting over three hours." She called me a doctor, but I am still a medical student. Sounds awkward but good.

The door opens almost as abruptly as it had closed. He looks at me with a stern but friendly expression. "Come on in." Shaking my hand and leading me into his office, he glances back at the secretary. "Bring in his file." And with that, slams the door behind him and takes a seat at his cluttered desk.

"What do you want to be when you grow up? A surgeon?" He doesn't give me time to answer. "Do you know what kind of internship program we have here? You are on call at the hospital every other night, but you work every night. On your nights off, you don't get home until ten or eleven, if you get home at all. Are you aware of that?"

"Yes sir."

"You have five years to do an internship and residency. That's not enough time, so you either tack on an extra two years or you work day and night for five years. That's the way we run it here; you work hard but you also get to operate. Do you like to operate?"

"Yes sir."

"Look at this." He reaches into a drawer and pulls out a small red paperback manual entitled *Surgery Handbook* and tosses it on his desk for me to pick up. "Look on page thirty-four. You'll see a list of operations performed by three interns last year. You won't find a list with as many cases anywhere in the country." The secretary hands him a folder with my name printed on the front. In it are letters of recommendation and the transcript of my grades for the first three years of medical school. That small folder represents college and medical school. My whole past is laid out before him and my entire future rests on his evaluation of my medical life up to this very moment. There is no way to convince him to accept me by sitting in his office and talking to him unless my past record is favorable. Never before have I felt the realization of the value of hard work over an extended period. All of the nights spent studying in medical school; any sacrifices I may have made; any hardships I have endured, all are wrapped up in the folder Dr. Eler is holding. That folder is analogous to the silk sutures tied to the refrigerator door handle. It is a priceless symbol. There is no amount of money I would take in exchange for those few pieces of paper he is reading.

Dr. Eler looks up from his desk. "Do you plan on general surgery, or a speciality?"

"I plan to go into general surgery, but also am interested in chest surgery." I become a little less tense, after the initial shock of actually saying a whole sentence to the man I have heard so much about.

"Did you apply for a straight surgery internship here?" he butts in.

"No sir, I applied for a mixed program with six months of surgery and the rest split between medicine and pediatrics. I had my interview this morning."

"You want to do a surgical residency here?"

"Yes sir, I certainly would like to plan in that direction."

"Then you want to do a straight surgical internship. I'll have to tear up your present application and you fill out a new one for a straight surgery before you leave here today."

The next few minutes go rapidly with a quick breakdown of the residency program; what to expect; what to tell my wife to expect. It is evident that I will be working more than I ever thought possible, and will not have much of a home life for the next five years—if I am accepted here. Not once in the conversation does Dr. Eler mention that I can have a spot in his program as an intern. I know the rules of the matching programs prohibit any agreements, written or verbal, prior to the matching data, but I think he could at least hint one way or the other. He is so straightforward and strictly business, I get no hint what his evaluation of me is.

At the end of the interview, we shake hands and I start making a new application. After looking at the choice of types of internship, I check the box beside "straight surgery." With this application, I know I am correct in my choice. After talking to Dr. Eler, there is no doubt about what I should do. Now, if he will only accept me.

I decide to take a rain check on making rounds. I am too excited to wait to tell Harriet about my three "wasted" interviews and my "golden" one with Dr. Eler.

"Well, why do you think I won't like it if you say it's such a good program? It sounds just like what you've been looking for," she says.

I hesitate to explain. "You know all the other places we've looked. Do you remember the interns are on every third night? Every third night is not so bad because if I were up all night, then I could sleep the next and have the third night free to do what we want." I explain the situation as best I can to make her understand how hard it is gong to be on her in case I get accepted for this program.

"I know you are leading up to something bad, but go ahead," she responds.

"Interns and residents are on every other night here. The bad part is that Dr. Eler says that even on our nights off we get home late and if everyone is busy, we may not get home at all."

Harriet makes a peculiar face, answering in disbelief: "How can they expect you to work like that. You can't operate without sleep. Anyone knows that."

"I'm sure we will get some sleep. Maybe not a lot, but at least enough to operate. Anyway, that's the way the program is run, and it looks like exactly what I need. It's like Dr. Eler said, I could go somewhere else to a seven year program and not have to work as hard, or even a five year program which is easier, but he thinks a surgeon ought to give every minute of those five years of his life to learning to become a surgeon. He feels its 'that' important, and I have to agree with him. The entire remaining years of practice are based on these next five years, and it is essential that I get a good base to work on." I really don't know if Harriet is listening, or thinking, or just staring out the front window of the car, but our conversation ends for some time.

Finally, she breaks the silence. "Why don't you try to get on here?"

I thought she would say something like that. She always has. I suppose she realized what she was getting into when we married.

"It will be better some day," I remind her now as I have so many times before.

As we head for home, I think back over the goal structure I see unfolding.

MAJOR GOAL: Complete surgical training
INTERMEDIATE GOAL: Find a good surgical residency training program
IMMEDIATE ACTION GOAL: Find a good mixed internship

I started out looking for a mixed internship. In all manner of reasoning, that was my immediate action goal. However, it ultimately was going to stand in the way of reaching my intermediate goal of a good surgical residency. So, the immediate action goal had to change to a straight surgery internship program in order to enhance getting a surgery residency program. Bingo—the opportunity door cracked open for the surgery program, and I had to be flexible enough to change my immediate action goal of a mixed internship to that of a straight surgery internship for the sake of reaching the intermediate goal of a good surgery resident program, and finally becoming a surgeon. Why was the opportunity easy for me to see and decision easy to make to change to a straight surgical program? There was only one answer. The compelling desire for my major goal is so strong, that anything related to the success of it comes easy. Sure, that's the secret. The stronger the desire for a goal, the easier it is to see the opportunities to enhance it and the easier the decision comes to change immediate action goals.

I feel good with this discovery of sureness in my decision to shoot for a straight surgery internship. My compelling desire to become a surgeon is so strong, any opportunity to enhance this goal becomes crystal clear; definite; without doubt.

We return home from our "vacation" and fill out the list on the matching program in order of preference as to where I want to do my internship. I seal the envelope, drop it in the mail, and try to forget the possibilities I have of getting my first choice. Nothing to do now but wait until December when the results are made known. In the meantime, I need to finish the summer job on surgery and prepare for the last year in medical school.

The first three months of the senior year pass quickly. This seems to be the easiest year so far because the pressure is off and I do not feel as compelled to study every working hour of the day. One thought keeps coming up; I wonder if I will get my choice of internship.

The big day arrives; December 6, and all the matches are fed into the computer. The senior class is called into the auditorium to receive the sealed envelopes from the matching program. The names are called in alphabetical order. Some open their envelope as soon as it is handed to them, others stick it in their pocket and walk right out of the auditorium to solitude where no one will know their results. There are shouts of joy from students who are matched with the hospitals of their choice; I see gloomy faces around, too. Evidently, they either did not get matched at all or are matched with their fourth or fifth choice.

I develop a case of butterflies as my name is called. I return to my seat with the white envelope and tear the end of it off, blow nervously into it to separate the enclosed letter from the edges and lift the all important statement out. "I know I can do the job if he will just let me try," I keep thinking to myself about Dr. Eler as I go through the ritual of removing the letter. At first, just a glance; I can read the whole letter later but I am sure my excited eyes can quickly find if I have been accepted by—yes! There it is! "The boss" is going to give me a chance to get into his program. I am one of sixteen interns hand-picked by him to work under his supervision. A lump comes to my throat. I can't laugh, can't talk, can't do anything except feel good all over. By simple mathematics of the program having sixteen interns and eight first year residents, I know only half of the interns he has accepted will end up in his residency program. But somehow I feel I can make the cutoff if only given the chance. Now, I have the chance.

I am so excited that I rush home to tell Harriet the good news. I can tell she is happy for me, but at the same time apprehensive about what lies ahead. However, neither of us has an inkling of what great excitement truly lies ahead of us in the next few months.

Time now seems to slow down and it seems as if school will last forever. Then suddenly an event happens that really wakes us up.

It is a cold and rainy night with the early March winds blowing the sheets of rain against the tin roof outside our bedroom window. Harriet and I are propped up in bed reading. She puts her magazine down and takes hold of my arm with both hands. "Do you know what I think?" She has a gleam in her eyes which means that there is no earthly way I can guess what's on her mind.

"I give up," I respond as I lay my book on the spread, happy for an excuse to quit studying for awhile.

"I think I'm pregnant."

"You think what!?"

"I think I'm pregnant, I made an appointment this afternoon to be checked Friday."

How can she be so calm about this? To just lie there and calmly tell me she thinks she's pregnant. Now it's my turn to be apprehensive.

"That's good. That's really good!" I hold her close as the rain continues to play its special symphony just for us—the three of us.

Life is becoming more exciting; internship approaching, surgical residency to look forward to . . . and a family.

Senior year continues to be an easy one consisting mostly of rotating on the subspecialities of surgery and medicine. It is while on these rotations I become aware of the true correlation between medicine and surgery; how most subspecialities in surgery have a corresponding subspeciality in medicine. There is renal medicine/urology surgery; pediatric medicine/pediatric surgery; gastroenterology/general surgery on the intestinal tract; pulmonary medicine/chest surgery; cardiology medicine/cardiac surgery. Each of these pairs of specialities goes hand in hand in treating the patient.

There is perpetual talk between the residents in medicine and the residents in surgery concerning which is more important in treating the patient—medicine or surgery. The medical residents say surgeons are just a bunch of technicians and that trained monkeys could do their jobs. In turn, the surgical residents reply that medicine consists of giving pills and when one pill doesn't work, they try another till the patient either gets well on his own or has to be cured by the knife. Occasional talk in this vein is good fun with some of the residents, but with others it is no laughing matter. As I rotate from one subspeciality to another, I realize that neither group of residents is correct; it takes the difficult years of learning on both sides to be able to treat the different patients.

Other than the subspecialities of medicine and surgery, I rotate through a few weeks of pediatric clinics, neurology, psychiatry and a few more one- to two-week rotations that are used only as an introduction to a particular branch of medicine.

By the end of May it is all over but the shouting. Graduation is near and no one is worrying about anything. We still have state boards to take, but it has been years since anyone failed the exam; anyway, we have been studying for four years and a few hours of cramming at this time will not change our true medical knowledge one iota.

Class rings cost too much. "I'll get one later when we have more money," I tell Harriet. I wouldn't wear it anyway; my wedding ring is enough trouble to take off every time I have to scrub for surgery.

We are fitted for graduation gowns, a few in the class even buy them. They are dashingly handsome with all the colors and velvet, but that remains low on the list of what I want to buy with the money I have. The gown is uncomfortable, but it does stir excitement just trying it on.

I have to check with the administration office to insure I'm not leaving any unattended matters; I leave a forwarding address for my grades to be sent. They hold little value any more. Medical school is behind and whether I will be accepted into Dr. Eler's residency program depends solely on how I do my internship, not on present grades.

Everyone in the class passes state boards, and the night of graduation arrives. As I sit awaiting all the preliminaries, I reflect on some of the basic thoughts. It is almost anticlimatic to four years of hard work. I am now a doctor, but why doesn't graduation mean more than it does. I look at the reality of the situation. I was partly a doctor the first day of medical school. I was more of a doctor when I started my first I.V. I was more of a doctor when I delivered my first baby and operated on a dog, and even more when I performed my first hernia operation. This fits with what I wrote years ago in my book. The definition of success: I am successful as long as I am working toward my major goal.

Many would say I became successful the day I graduated from medical school. I say I became successful the day I began to work toward medical school and remained a successful individual throughout the training period.

The realization comes to light. The success of becoming a doctor is no more than the accumulation of a series of immediate action goals. I haven't realized it until now, but the really important factors of success have been those day by day actions. I can look ahead to studying surgery with the proper importance placed on the daily immediate action goals as I am confronted by them.

One does not have to wait until attainment of a goal to be, feel, or appear successful. As a matter of fact, I am already getting a slight hint of what it will be like when I become a surgeon because as of this date, I will apply myself one hundred percent to becoming a surgeon.

I reflect back over the past four years. A lot has happened; marriage started, medical school completed. There is no way anyone could have told me what school would be like. There is no way to describe the odor of the cadavers that first year. No one could possibly explain the hidden emotional strain of the first examination. The first delivery will always remain a milestone toward actually becoming a physician. When it all began, I decided to set goals but there were hundreds of times that I had to act immediately in order to acomplish a certain project. It has not been as easy as setting a goal and doing it. One goal has built upon another in such a fashion that the process becomes a life pattern after awhile; a second nature sense about getting jobs done. I have come to know what it means "a job once begun is never complete until it's done." So many times I have read 97 out of a 100 page reading assignment and wanted to quit without reading those last three pages. So many times have I wanted to not review some material the second or third time. It has been a real urge to leave those loose ends dangling. But I have found that the last two to three percent effort makes all the difference, because most students will not make the last effort. I also came to realize that most of the time that extra effort does not make any difference at all at the time but sooner or later it does matter. There is no way to pick and choose those times when it will make a difference.

So, I look forward to this coming year as an intern in a different way than I looked forward to the first year of medical school. I realize so much more now than then. I realize there will be many uncontrollables, many instances where I won't know what to do. But I also realize that I will somehow work through it. The goal structure has worked thus far and I am certain it will continue to do so. Internship year is a big unknown, a very decisive time in my life. I know my future training in surgery, and ultimately what type of surgeon I become, rests on my performance this year. I am going to give it my best.

Part II
INTERNSHIP

INTERNSHIPS AND RESIDENCIES begin July 1 of each year, but I have been instructed to appear one week early for orientation. Harriet and I find an unfurnished apartment near the hospital, shop the used furniture stores, buy only a bed and a table with four chairs. We officially move in, and I am ready to begin the year of internship.

The first few days are routine, learning where everything is located, reviewing the charts of patients we will be picking up as our own, and meeting the residents we will work with. As with any orientation, they could have told us in one day what it takes five to do—but the big day finally arrives! July 1. The past interns gleefully become residents, and the night scut work they did for a year now becomes the work of the new interns.

They seem so confident. I wonder if I can possibly be that way after just one year. I think how much difference one year can make; right now I'm not sure I can start an I.V., and the interns leaving seem to have no trouble in completely caring for the patients. The job seems too big. We look at how much these last day interns have learned and to look at what I know right now places insurmountable odds against me. It is like looking at a bricklayer just beginning to lay bricks for a fifteen story building.

My mind eases and a relaxed half smile comes to my lips. That's the secret. It lies with the bricklayer. He does it one brick at a time. I won't look one year down the road. I'll look at today's brick and make it one brick at a time. After all, buildings get built this way.

Here at the medical center, there is a teaching type conference each week day and two on Saturday. The ones during the week are hour long sessions that include the joint efforts of the medicine department and the surgery department, but the two on Saturday are limited to surgery. Dr. Eler, as chief of surgery, is in complete charge; his true personality comes streaming forth as strong and forceful as a Colorado River rapid proving its supremacy to the rest of nature.

"Grand Rounds" is the title given the first Saturday conference, and it is held in the hospital auditorium. As we enter the room, a handout sheet is given to each of us and on it is the topic of the day: Carcinoma of the Colon. Twenty references are listed; each a journal article for quick reference in the future to review the next time we scrub on a colon case. This sheet represents another example of Dr. Eler's organization.

The staff surgeons, as well as several private surgeons from town, line the front row in the auditorium. Dr. Eler stands at the podium and stares at some papers he is holding. He appears to be staring at the papers, but by focusing all my attention on what he is doing I notice he intermittently glances at the auditorium clock hanging on the wall. He is not looking at his papers at all, he is watching the time. Exactly when the red second hand signifies nine o'clock sharp, Dr. Eler begins talking and the conference is started—punctually.

Exactly one hour later, he rises from his seat, interrupts the discussion and announces: "The conference is over. The interns and residents will now go to the classrooms on the second floor for the 'Morbidity and Mortality' conference. Students are *not* invited."

"Does he always run things this way?" I ask the resident beside me.

"Oh yes. He even locks the doors to the lecture room at seven o'clock when he is lecturing to the students, and if any of them are one second late, they may as well have stayed home in bed because he won't let them in. You get used to being on time around here. As a matter of fact, we had better get over to the 'M & M' conference. That is one meeting to which you don't want to be late.

"M & M" conference is the slang attached to the Morbidity and Mortality conference which consists of discussing all the complications and deaths that occurred during the week on surgery. This is noted to be the best teaching tool Dr. Eler uses in his residency program. Everyone has to list any complication or death that occurred on his patients during the preceeding week and be prepared to discuss it with complete knowledge of the subject. A simple complication may require several hours reading and reviewing of the subject in surgical journals. It is well known, however, that no matter how well a resident prepares himself for the meeting, the last question asked by Dr. Eler will be unanswerable. He may ask only two questions before he surpasses the resident's knowledge of the subject; it may take him twenty questions; but there will always be that end point where he proves the resident's incomplete knowledge of surgery.

The first M & M lasts until one-thirty Saturday afternoon. I quickly realize Dr. Eler's compulsive punctuality plays no role in deciding when the M & M conference is concluded. It ends only when Dr. Eler asks the last unanswerable question of the last intern or resident.

After driving home, I think over the M & M conference. It has to be the epitome of the two best methods of learning; the "I have to go through myself" experience, and the "I don't have to go through myself" experience. The more I can learn from the complications of another intern or resident, the less chance I have of having the same complications with a patient. I pull the *Goal's Rule Book* from my pocket, and look back at what I have written while on pediatrics as a student: There are two basic methods of learning: The "I have to go through myself" experience and the "I don't have to go through myself' experience. Learn as many "don't have to's" as possible.

The year of internship will be split between several types of surgery: urology, neurosurgery, gynecological surgery, orthopedics, emergency room and general surgery. The first month will take me through the teachings of orthopedics.

The first night, I am placed "on call." This entails completing the work to be done on the ward and sleeping in the hospital by the phone in case there is any problem on the orthopedic service that the nurse may want me to handle. It is ironic. My first night as an intern, and I am supposed to know how to handle any problem that may come up during the night on any of the twenty patients.

My pulse jumps to at least one hundred and forty each time the phone rings, and I remain so excited after each call, it takes forever to get back to sleep. I hate to be called, but there is a sense of satisfaction that I now have had some responsibility as an M.D., not "just" a student any more. I know absolutely no more now than I did as a senior medical student one month ago, but now it is different, I am an intern and expected to know how to handle problems that come up. I think people will do what is expected of them, and I know it will be only a matter of time before I begin to accomplish the expectations of every intern. It is just so awkward answering the phone. I hope my learning is not long on coming.

The third day on the service, I am baptized into my first real surgical procedure since becoming an intern when I am given a patient who needs an amputation. Mr. Butler was previously admitted for an operation on his arteries to save his leg but refused surgery at that time. It is now his fate to have the leg removed, and I am chosen to be the surgeon to perform the procedure. Dr. Bowen is head of the department of orthopedic surgery and will assist me in this, my first major operation.

I hurry to Mr. Butler's room as soon as I am notified of his admission to the hospital. He has a gangrenous right foot with the odor of dead flesh and infection. He is a gentle, easygoing man, who does not reveal any pain from his dead foot. On the contrary, he only smiles and nods as I examine him.

"Why didn't you let them operate when you were in here before?" I ask sympathetically. I start my history taking and physical examination in preparation for his amputation scheduled in the morning. His wife sits in the corner of the room saying nothing. By looking at her clothes, it is easy to see that the Butlers are not from an affluent background. She wears a thin cotton print dress with most of the buttons missing and held together with a combination of safety pins. Her shoes are all but worn out, the sides split down to large bunions on each big toe. A little trickle of tobacco juice leaks out the corner of her mouth, and the lower lip protrudes where she has stashed away a morning's supply of snuff. Mr. and Mrs. Butler are typical of the charity cases on which we operate. They are just plain old mountain folk, salt of the earth types who have worked hard all their lives and very seldom sought medical help until they were almost dead, or in such a condition as Mr. Butler—nothing to do but amputate.

"Thought I could tough it out and get better, but it only got worse. Can you do anything for it, Doc?"

"Well, I'm afraid we can't do an operation to *save* your leg, but we can amputate to keep the infection from getting into your system and making you sick all over," I explain. He takes this at face value, asks no more questions, shows no remorse at not having had the operation on his arteries to save his leg two years before, and does not inquire as to what he should expect from his vascular disease in the future. Neither does his wife ask any questions nor change her expression when I mention "amputation." This is all new to them. They never went to such medical facilities prior to the opening of this hospital. There were hospitals around, but they had never seen fit to enter the doors other than on an occasional visit to a sick friend. I don't know much more to say to them other than explain the operation and tell them what to expect after the surgery.

"You'ns ain't gonna bury his leg in the ground, aire ya?" His wife gives me the first indication of acceptance of me as a surgeon. "They cut Uncle Charlie's leg off and buried hit in the ground and the ants got to hit and Uncle Charlie said he could feel them things acrawlin' all over his leg, even tho he didn't have hit no more."

The complaints of ants crawling on Uncle Charlie's leg is referred to medically as "phantom pain." Many patients with amputations continue to "feel" the leg and to have different aches and pains related to that part which is no longer with them. The reason for this is that the nerve in the leg is an extension of the large nerve in the thigh. This nerve still sends sensations to the brain, and the brain interprets these as coming from the foot, or the leg, or from wherever the nerve impulse used to originate. The vague, tingling sensations occasionally feel like ants or bugs crawling around. I am sure Mrs. Butler will never accept this explanation.

I don't know what to tell her. I have never thought about what is done with the extremities after they are amputated. I assume they are just buried—in the ground. I surely can't tell her that though.

"I'll make sure it isn't buried in the ground," I reassure her as I make a quick exit from the room. "We will be back this afternoon in case you think of any more questions concerning the operation." At least Dr. Bowen will be on rounds with me and perhaps he can answer any questions better than I.

I am off for the night at six and head for the library. I check out the large surgical atlas: *Techniques in Surgery, General and Abdominal.* "Amputation, supracondylar, right, 610–617." I find the operation in the index and flip to page 610. On one page are step-by-step illustrations of the procedure, and the adjacent page has a description and explanation of each drawing. I wade through the pages of drawings of muscles, arteries, veins, and nerves I will encounter as I cut across the thigh. I haven't looked at them since my first month in medical school. I guess I had better learn all the branches of arteries that pass through the area; Dr. Bowen will probably ask that also. The more I study, the more I realize how much I have to re-learn. Dr. Bowen made a special point to the residents on evening rounds that he was going to help me, since it was my first amputation, and they could watch. To me, that means they can watch him drill me to the wall with questions about the procedure.

There is so much to learn. I decide the best approach will be to write it down. Step by step. Write it down. Where do I cut through the skin? Write it down. What is the first muscle I will encounter? Write it down. What is the next instrument I will ask for? Write it down. There seems to be something almost magical about writing it down. Soon, I have the entire operation written down from my first cut to the last stitch.

By eleven P.M., I can do the operation in my mind. I can see my hands working. I can see the anatomy. I know the next step. I know the next instrument I need and can ask for it. There is no doubt whatsoever—I can do the operation. I have already performed it three times tonight in my mind.

We have an eight o'clock spot on the schedule, which means I am to be in the operating room at seven-thirty to get things rolling. Intravenous fluids have to be started, Mr. Butler's leg shaved, the operative site scrubbed for ten minutes, and I have to scrub my hands for ten minutes before beginning the operation. At five to eight, everything is going as planned. I am in the midst of scrubbing Mr. Butler's leg when Dr. Bowen enters the room. We are ready to begin the operation at eight-ten.

"What kind of skin incisions are you going to make?" Dr. Bowen asks.

"I thought I would make the anterior flap from just above the patella to five centimeters above the femoral condyle."

"O.K., that sounds reasonable enough. Go to it."

The first pass of my knife goes through skin, the little bit of fat beneath the skin, and into the fascia covering the muscle.

"You cut through the fascia! That's too deep. You want to cut through the skin, then pull the skin up his leg and cut the fascia at a higher level, then pull both skin and fascia even higher and cut the muscle. Finally, pull the muscle up and saw the bone at even a higher level. You want to make an inverted cone out of the wound, so that the bone will be well padded and not sticking out into the open when you finish. Now, cut the fascia a little higher, the correct way."

He has just gone through the whole operation in one sentence. I know all that. Just because I had a little adrenalin flowing, I cut too deeply. I know the steps of the operation but I did cut deep, so there is no use saying anything; just make another incision through the fascia a little higher and keep going.

"The first thing you want to do is find big red and big blue, isn't it?" Dr. Bowen appears to be having a good time, even though I am not particularly enjoying it. I feel he is toying with me just to put on a performance in front of the residents. However, he is one of the best teachers in the program, and I know I will learn from this experience.

"Big red and big blue," I think to myself. "Surely he can't be referring to the femoral artery and vein, with no respect to formal anatomy. I guess he is; that's the next step in the operation."

"Yes sir," I reply.

"Well, dig them out and tie them off before you cut someone with that big knife you're flashing around.

I lay the knife down and ask for some scissors and pickups— dissect down between the mucles and find the femoral artery, vein, and nerve. I clean the tissues around each and ligate them with silk sutures. I place one suture high, one low and cut between so no blood will spill into the wound from either direction.

"What's your next move? Look's like you're doing all right so far."

I think back to the night before. Here it comes. I've got to name all the muscles as I cut through each one. I'm not sure I can remember well enough to name them without hesitating between some. "I am going to start by cutting the vastus medialis of the quadriceps femoris." I begin to spill back what I memorized last evening.

"Now wait a minute," Dr. Bowen breaks in, stops the entire operation, and leans forward just in front of my face. "You are not going to stand here and name each muscle of the thigh are you? You don't think you will be able to identify each one of those as you cut through them, do you? If you did, we would be here all day. Now, what you are really going to do is cut all the *front* muscles and then cut all the *back* muscles and then saw the bone in two. Now, isn't that what you are really going to do?"

"Yes sir . . . essentially that's all I'm going to do."

I can't help but feel a small amount of aggravation at this point. I think of all the reviewing I did last night. "Big red, big blue, front muscles, back muscles"; he's got to be kidding—this is an amputation on a human, not a frog. He makes it sound like I am a mechanic changing spark plugs. I keep these thoughts to myself but find it difficult to realize he is only trying to get a practical point across. On the other hand, the residents are enjoying his comments enormously.

I slice the muscle bundles down to the bone and begin to saw with the little hand saw orthopedic surgeons use.

"Haven't you ever sawed a metal pipe in two before?" Dr. Bowen interrupts. "Act like you want to get through the bone today, not tomorrow. You would never make an orthopedic surgeon sawing like that."

I double my rhythm with the saw—just like cutting a metal pipe. I finish sawing and fill the marrow with wax since it is soft and will continue to ooze blood if not plugged. I suture the front flap of muscles to the back flap and stick a rubber drain in the wound to allow any blood that may accumulate to escape out the drain instead of being trapped inside the wound.

As we put the dressing on, I ask Dr. Bowen, "What happens to the leg after we send it to pathology?"

"They burn it," he replies. "Why?"

"I was just wondering . . . just wondering."

After writing post-operative orders on the chart and taking the patient to the recovery room, I now have time to be alone and rehash the events of the morning. There is a certain accomplishment in life each time we do something for the first time. I have mixed feelings about accomplishing my first operation as an intern. It went well but not as I envisioned it last night. Everything had gone perfectly in my mind while I thought through each step of the procedure as I lay in bed before going to sleep; could see myself speeding through the operation and Dr. Bowen standing amazed at how well I knew the anatomy and how quick and sure my hands moved from one step to the next. I could see him telling me how well I had done at the completion of the procedure. Now that it's over, the point that stands out in my mind most is the fact he didn't like the way I used a saw. Nevertheless, I have used my goal structure to its fullest. I have conquered my first surgical test successfully.

MAJOR GOAL: Become a surgeon
INTERMEDIATE GOAL: Perform first case successfully
IMMEDIATE ACTION GOAL: Action. Study. Write it down.
Do the operation in my mind. See my hands working. See the

anatomy. Know the next step. Learn the right way to use a saw. Write it down until I can operate in my mind just as fast as I can write.

The *Goal's Rule Book* is working.

I must accept the fact of having to jump the hurdle of "firsts" many more times through the internship year. The one jump I have dreaded for two weeks is again announced: "Code 500, Seven I.C.U. Code 500, Seven I.C.U." This is the code used in the hospital to notify all doctors of a cardiac arrest at a specific location. Whenever announced, all available doctors are to rush to the scene to begin resusitation; revive the patient. This time, the call is for the intensive care unit.

I take off for the stairwell, begin the long run to the seventh floor; the elevator takes too long and besides, there is no way to hurry once on an elevator stopping at each floor. As I take two steps at a time rushing as fast as I can, I become aware that my mind is doing two things: it is making my body move to the scene as rapidly as possible, but also hoping I don't get there before anyone else. What would I do if I were the first to arrive? There would be four or five nurses already with the patient; within seconds, the "crash cart" with all the necessary drugs and items needed would be rolled in by two technicians; the electrocardiogram cart would be wheeled in by yet another technician, and two other nurses would plug in the defibrillator paddles and stand ready in case the heart needed an electrical shock to stimulate it into action. All these individuals begin working on the patient until the arrival of one person who takes charge when he comes into the room—the first doctor to arrive at the scene.

I don't want to be the first to arrive. But, if I do only things I want to do, I will never reach my major goal. I am sure no other intern wants to be the first to arrive either, but I must push myself to do things I don't particularly like to do in order to reach my goals. It is the immediate action goals that I don't like but realize the necessity.

I know the reason I don't want to be the first to arrive. It's because I don't know exactly what to do. I know some of the things that have to be done initially, but there are a hundred different diverging paths that may need to be taken on any given patient, and I haven't yet gained the experience it takes to run the show from beginning to end. It can only be a matter of time before I do arrive first and will be called on to handle the situation, but I do not want that time to be now. I want to learn some more before I have to handle a "Code 500."

I burst into the I.C.U., my mind ready to work at one hundred percent capacity if needed. The chief resident is present and already working on reviving the patient. I am relieved for the moment. Now, I must observe *everything* he does and commit it to memory, not the kind of memory I used in college to memorize an organic chemistry formula for a test, but the kind of memory that is stored in the computer mind for quick, practical recall at a crucial time. I have to start filling up each of the hundred diverging paths of how to treat the patient, and the sooner I get them filled, the more comfortable I will feel, and the better off the patient will be.

I take notice of each drug he uses, when he uses it, the dosage. I watch him feel for the pulse, eye the electrocardiogram, inject medication into the vein; then into the heart. I listen as he tells the nurse how much to charge the defibrillating paddles, as he tells another nurse to inject some I.V. medications. I watch, I listen. I am aware only of what the chief resident is saying and doing, block out all other conversation of the nurses, junior resident, technicians. This, I must learn how to do firsthand. There is no book written that can tell a doctor how to handle a Code 500. Only observation . . . experience . . . doing, can ever teach me this portion of becoming a doctor. This definitely falls into a "I have to go through myself" experience. I again realize I must do things others don't particularly like to do in order to reach my goals.

The patient is revived, and the anitclimax of routine patient care prevails once again. I leave the unit and make ready for morning chores.

Another day of internship passes. Another, and another. Dr. Bowen is the best teacher of surgery I have ever worked with and I would like to spend more time with him, but my schedule calls for me to spend the next month on pediatric surgery.

There is so much to learn, no way my mind can conceive of doing big surgery when it does not even know how to do an appendectomy; it boggles the mind to even think about acquiring that much knowledge. There is only one solution to the problem: "One stitch at a time." First, I will learn the basis of cutting and sewing, then start putting them together in the form of an amputation, a hernia, an appendectomy, a gall bladder, a stomach, a lung, a heart. That will be the system; one stitch at a time.

The service is small, just a first year resident, Len Stewart, and me. I want to learn to do two types of cases while on this rotation—hernias and appendectomies. There are always plenty of hernias scheduled during the month, but the appendectomies seem to come in spurts and entire months have gone by without a single "appie" coming in.

Two weeks pass. I have performed seven hernia operations, but I begin worrying about not having the experience of the "first appendix" under my belt. It is supposed to be an easy operation, but until I do one I have no way to measure the difficulty for certain. As with so many aspects of life, there is no good gauge with which to measure the difficulty of a particular operation. On an arbitrary scale of one to ten, one surgeon may list an appendectomy as a "one." Another surgeon may be technically poor and after having several difficult appendix operations, may list it as a "five." This same surgeon may develop competency as his years of surgery progress and he may change the rating back down to a "two." Again, some surgeons tend to overestimate the difficulty of a procedure, while others underestimate it. The only true rating I can place on any given operation can come only after I have performed it. Thus, the fact that I have not done one dangles in the forefront of my mind daily.

Two "possible appendix" cases come into the emergency room by week's end, but both prove to be intestinal flu. I am scheduled to be off for the weekend but instruct Len to give me a ring if an appendix turns up.

The phone rings at one-thirty Sunday morning. I am sleeping so soundly that Harriet has to wake me to answer it.

"Len here."

"Yes, Len; what's up?"

"Your appendix came in about half an hour ago. Still want to do it?"

"It will take about fifteen minutes to get there, but don't start cutting without me."

Harriet looks at me in disbelief. "You aren't on call. How can they expect you to come in when you aren't even on call?"

I am sure there is no way to explain it to her. "Look, this will only take an hour or so and I'll be back home before you really get

— 91 —

back to sleep." In the few short weeks of my internship I have quickly come to realize that no matter how much a wife may love her husband, no matter how much she tries to think like him, no matter how much she tries to want what he wants, the feelings of the intern and wife are different. Harriet wants me to obtain the surgical training I desire, wants me to work hard at it, and to obtain the goal I have set for myself; however, she also wants me at home some of the time and awake at least part of the time I am there. There is no way for me to convey my reasoning to her. I, too, like to come home and would rather be awake than asleep, but the desire to become a surgeon keeps reminding me I must take advantage of every opportunity that comes my way.

What makes this desire? What makes desire a compulsion? What makes up compelling desire in someone? Why is it so strong, my desire to become a surgeon, that I will get up in the middle of the night and go operate? I don't know. But it is there and it's growing stronger as I feed it with completed immediate action goals.

Harriet turns over in bed. She is upset. Not because I am going to work the rest of the night; she will still get a good night's sleep. The problem comes in the morning. Tomorrow afternoon. The one day in two weeks I have to spend with my pregnant wife, I will be sleeping. It is not fair to her and she knows it. It is not fair to our marriage. Internship is a strong competition for my time. There is really nothing for me to say. I realize what she is thinking and why she is reacting the way she is. I know I should say something, but I don't. I dress with the light off. Maybe that will say something. I ease out of the bedroom as if she has fallen back to sleep and quietly close the door to the apartment and head for the hospital.

The patient is still in the emergency room when I arrive. They are finishing a case on general and we have the operating room next.

Len is in the chart room sipping coffee. "The patient is in room three. Go see what you think; didn't do a rectal, saved that for you," Len laughs and returns to his coffee.

There is a little boy and his mother in the room. He appears to be about eight years old. He lies very still on the examining table with his knees pulled under him, cheeks flushed with fever. His face remains expressionless as he rolls his eyes up to meet mine.

"When did the pain start?" I ask his mother as I gently roll him over onto his back and pull his shirt up to his chest.

"Started last night about this time," she replies. "Thought it was something he ate, so I gave him some stomach medicine, which helped for awhile, but this morning he started vomiting. He got worse, so I thought I'd better bring him in."

I look back into the boy's face. "What's your name?"

"Billy." He speaks quietly. He is shy. He has never been in a hospital, never been so dependent on a stranger like me.

He points to an exact spot which is typical for appendicitis, located in the right lower quadrant of the abdomen.

"Now Billy, I am going to push over here on your left side, and when I lift my hand up, you tell me where it hurts."

I push on the lower left portion of his abdomen, let up, and Billy grimaces immediately. "It hurts in the same place," he says, pointing to the spot on his right side.

"I want to do one more thing, Billy and then I'll leave you alone. I want to put my finger in your rectum and feel around." I push my finger into his rectum and point toward the left side. "I know that's uncomfortable but is there much pain when I push on that side."

Billy only shakes his head, no.

"What about now?" I push on the right side and Billy lets out a little whimper of pain.

"That makes it hurt again" he says in a quivering voice.

I withdraw my finger, turn to his mother and explain that I think he does have appendicitis and will need surgery as soon as we can get a room.

"Should I have brought him in sooner, doctor?"

"I think you got him here soon enough. He'll be sick for a few days but he will do all right." Of course, it really would have been better if she had brought him in twenty-four hours sooner but how was she to know. Besides, she has enough on her mind for the time being, without reprimanding her for bringing him in late.

I walk back to the chart room. "Looks like you found me a classic one, Len."

"I thought that would be nice for your first one," he gives a big smile. "Give me a call when you get him in the room and ready to be put to sleep. I'm going to catch a few winks in the resident's office while we wait."

A good half hour passes before the O.R. calls for the patient, and another half hour goes by before the anesthesiologist is ready to put him to sleep. I wake Len about a quarter to four and tell him we are ready to begin.

This is the first time I have ever entered the abdominal cavity on a patient; only in dog surgery have I operated inside the abdomen. I cut through the skin and subcutaneous tissue down to muscle, start dissecting out the different layers and Len interrupts me. "Don't take all night just getting down to the appendix. You don't need to open each muscle separately; just push a clamp down to the peritoneum and spread."

I give it a try and am surprised at how quick and easy it is to go through the muscles. Len places two retractors into the wound and pulls the muscles apart, giving me an area about the size of my fist to work in. As I cut through the peritoneal lining of the abdominal cavity, pus extrudes into the wound. He has a ruptured appendix! He waited too long to come to the hospital, and now the operation will be prolonged and much more difficult to perform. After much digging around, I locate the appendix and remove it, wash out the abdomen with saline and place a drain into the area where all the pus was. I close the wound around the drain and tape the dressing in place.

We roll the patient to his room and make sure he is waking from anesthesia before talking with his mother about the operation.

It is six o'clock before I crawl back into bed at home. Harriet looks lonely lying on her side sleeping. I stare into the faintly lighted room as a new day is breaking. I resolve to stay awake today and spend time with Harriet. I will make myself stay awake today. I drift off to sleep, having the satisfaction of not only taking out my first appendix, but of taking out a ruptured appendix—a much more difficult case.

The routine of being an intern begins again Monday morning at five thirty. Harriet cooks me breakfast and makes a lunch. I am barely awake; I didn't nap at all yesterday afternoon.

Three nights later I am awakened by the nurse from the pediatric intensive care unit telling me the patient Len operated on today has a temperature of 103 degrees. I drag myself up to the unit to do a "fever check." I am not sure of the rationale for all my actions, but it is a combination of checks that all interns do when a patient develops a fever. I order a urinalysis to check for kidney infection—normal; draw blood for a complete blood count to see if the white count is elevated indicating the body is fighting an acute infection—negative; make the patient spit up some sputum to look at under the microscope to see if I can find any bacteria. I spend one and a half hours doing the fever check and still don't know what's causing it. I order an aspirin suppository and return to my room. I hate doing work like that. Just like a machine: get up, draw blood, check urine, look at sputum, give aspirin and go back to bed. I haven't found anything positive in a fever check, but it is expected when any patient who spikes a temperature of over 101.

Next morning on rounds, I discuss the patient with Len and tell him of my dilemma with routine checks.

"Who told you to do fever checks? I didn't." Len surprises me with his sarcastic reply.

"It's something all the interns do."

"I didn't when I was an intern," Len replies authoritatively.

"How will you ever find the cause of the fever if you don't do fever checks?" Two minutes ago I was ready to argue against doing such checks and now that Len lets me know he doesn't do them, I turn and take the defensive for doing the checks. I need to know the reasoning against doing them if I am ever to learn a good argument.

"Simple. If a patient develops a fever the night after surgery, it is coming from his lungs. If you would spend five minutes making the patient cough instead of an hour getting a fever check done, his temp would be down to normal by morning. Ninety-nine percent of surgical fevers come the first night after surgery, and if you remember to make them cough, you have half the battle licked. The second time period a post-op patient gets a fever is five days after surgery. You don't need to do a fever check—you need to look for an abscess. It will probably be in the wound, and if it is not there, it is wherever you operated. It is as simple as that. A first day fever needs coughing and a fifth day fever needs draining. Don't waste your time waiting for blood cultures. Go ahead and treat what's causing the fever." Len acts almost disgusted with my hour and a half effort last night.

I benefit, however, doubly from this experience. First, I know how to treat post-op fevers; secondly, I won't waste my time doing "routine" anythings. If I don't understand why I am doing something, I will ask until I find out the reasoning behind doing it. I will either find out the "whys" of post-operative care or find a better way of doing it. My biggest gain from the whole encounter is the fact that from now on, I will avoid practicing medicine the way everybody else does simply for the reason that "everybody else does it that way."

By the end of the rotation, I have three more appendectomies to place on my "gauge," as well as nine hernias. It has been a rewarding month; I feel more like a surgeon every day.

As the weeks pass, I begin to notice Melvin Slusher, a third year resident whom I consider the most intelligent resident in the program. As a result of reading every chance he gets, he knows most of the numbers and facts about the different surgical diseases. I respect his knowledge and admire him for it. We have not rotated on the same service together yet, but for some reason he picks me out of the rest of the interns to feed advice on how to "make it" in a competitive program.

Just after starting the third month of internship, Melvin and I start an informal discussion while having a cup of coffee at two in the morning after his finishing an emergency laparotomy and my finishing all my scut work for the night.

"Internship and residency are one big game played by yourself and your cohorts," Melvin says as he stretches out on the sofa in the resident's office. "There are sixteen interns in your group and only three chief resident spots in the program. Face it. Only three of you are going to make it to the top spot, and you have to figure a way to be a little better than anyone else at your level if you really want to make it in a competitive program. Every morning, every intern makes rounds at six-thirty with their resident, don't they? Half the interns in the program come running down to the operating room late just because they have work to be done on the ward before they make rounds. My advice is get up a half-hour earlier, get that scut work done and out of the way before the resident ever gets there. Then, you can go on to the operating room on time, or even early, and get the patient ready for surgery. You will stick out head and shoulders above the rest.

"Everyone needs some 'getting ahead' time, some time that one spends getting ahead of everyone else. Usually, this time is best found before everyone else gets up in the mornings. You remember that. Do more than just what is expected of you."

I thank him for his advice and check my notebook to make sure I haven't left any work undone.

"All done." I slam the book shut and bid Melvin goodnight.

"Wait a minute." He stares at me. "Let me see that scut book."

He glances over my work list. "I can't believe it. I don't believe you ever get your work done. No wonder you are still up at two in the morning. I am going to give you some advice that will be worth a month's paycheck to you, probably two months on your pay scale. You wrote that work list down this morning as it came to mind, didn't you? Then you didn't change it at all, did you? And you carried each out and checked it off your list in haphazard order, didn't you?"

All I can do is nod affirmatively. I don't see anything wrong so far.

"O.K. Here it is, the best advice you will ever get from me. After you write your list every morning, rewrite it in order of most importance to be done, then do the most important first, while you are still fresh. By the end of the day, all the important work is done and you are left with the less important tasks which don't drain you mentally. You can complete them quickly and get to bed. It will save you at least an hour a day. Use half of that time to get up early and you still come out with thirty minutes extra sleep."

If Melvin considers this the best advice he will ever give me, I'll do it. I thank him and head for bed although I am not particularly sleepy. Before turning out the light, I add two more rules to the goal's book: 1. Get ahead of others—Do more than is expected of me. 2. Write daily chores down in order of importance. I turn out the light, lie back and stare at the now black ceiling, and steal a few minutes of quiet time from Dr. Eler and his regime before dropping off to sleep. He will never know that I reserve a time I can think about anything I want. I think of non-surgery, of the outdoors, that of which I have temporarily been robbed, of mountain climbing, running a river, a hike in the Grand Canyon, a swim in the ocean— anything but surgery. I must make full use of my little secret closet of time, because so many nights only seconds pass between lying down and falling off to sleep; even as I fight to stay awake and travel with my thoughts.

I just fall into a sound sleep when I hear the phone ringing. "Good morning, it's five-thirty . . . don't go back to sleep now." The operator gives humorous advice that I can do without at five-thirty in the morning.

I hang up the phone, force myself to slide my feet to the floor and sit on the side of the bed, using knees to prop up elbows which in turn support my face resting in outreached fingers. "I can't do it," I think to myself. "I can't possibly start getting up thirty minutes earlier every morning." I continue to sit and contemplate my possible future and try to figure exactly how important Melvin said it was to get up and get started before anyone else.

I make it to the bathroom, flip on the light and stare at a blank face in the mirror as I rest against the sink. I do not know how long I stand looking in the mirror, but I do experience the same sensation in my eyelids that I have just before going to sleep . . . once closed, seconds pass before I can reopen them. Each blink, a miniature nap.

"O.K., I'll go along with you." I speak to the image in the mirror agreeing to make the early rising a practice plus organizing my list of work for the day. After all, my life is just one big habit of internship, so I might as well add two more habits to it. Especially after making my number one rule as an intern: Whenever a *positive* decision is made, never consider changing it; whenever a *negative* decision is reached, reconsider it after a full night's sleep.

I try this new system of starting earlier and organizing my work list and am astonished at how much better the whole day goes if I know I have not left something undone on the ward while being tied up all day in the operating room. With this new outlook, I begin to like internship more every day. Melvin was right. For the first time, I feel I am moving ahead of many of the interns. But best of all, I am finishing the scut work earlier and earlier. I become much more proficient at my chores of restarting I.V.s, changing dressings, drawing blood, writing a history and physical on the charts of the new patients admitted, making sure blood is in the blood bank for patients who have surgery the following morning, getting the pre-op patients to sign their operative permits, checking the chest x-rays on patients scheduled for surgery, removing sutures from patients who are to be discharged the following day, making post-operative patients cough after surgery by injecting saline into their tracheas, and attempting to read about the operations we will be scrubbing on the next day. I can't thank Melvin enough for his sound advice.

As time passes, I find myself referring more and more to the *Goal's Rule Book*. Internship becomes a true reality although my family life has suffered. Time at home is almost nil. I look forward to the time I can be at home more. It is time for Harriet to deliver. I am ready psychologically to have a child. I don't care whether it's a boy or girl, just so it's not like one of those Pinewood children I worked with on pediatrics in med school. I am not sure I am ready to have a child time wise. I will not get to spend any time with him or her for the next five years. Is it right to go ahead and start a family when there is so much demand on my time? How will it affect children to have basically only one parent for five years? There is no other way to do it. Harriet is going to have to carry the load competely. I have to depend on her for this. Right now she looks like she is going to split wide open if she doesn't go ahead and deliver soon.

Five o'clock in the morning, Harriet phones the on-call room at the hospital. She is having labor pains. Eighteen hours pass and she delivers—a boy, seven pounds, four ounces. I celebrate by going to bed and sleeping four straight hours without being called. I plan to live at the hospital in the on-call room until they are released from the hospital.

As far as time off, this is a bad time for me to become a father because I start neurosurgery in three days. But it is such an exciting time! He is such a small thing. We name him Ben. Both my grand-fathers were named Ben. It is difficult to believe. We actually are parents. Harriet lets me hold him but it feels so awkward; I'm afraid he will bend in the wrong places. I've held babies before but this one is so different. I hate to start neurosurgery, mainly because it is so time consuming. But I must come back down to earth and get back to work.

Time always allows the inevitable to happen, and before the newness of being a father wears off, the three days pass, and I am once more divorced from my wife and married to a new surgery rotation. The first few days of any rotation are unbelievable, but this one is especially difficult. I must learn quickly what the neuro-surgeons expect of me. I must learn twenty patients who are already on the service and work up the three new patients just admitted since I am the sole intern on neurosurgery. I will be on call every night. It appears impossible, but I feel confident time will prove its point once more, and I will develop new "time plans" to save valuable seconds, minutes, and even hours during the working day, and I will face this new rotation one stitch at a time, and I will survive.

*   *   *

During the first week we operate on several brain tumors and place several shunts in hydrocephalic babies. The cerebrospinal fluid, which continuously flows through the cavities of the brain and around the spinal cord, is blocked in these babies, and as the fluid builds up inside the brain, pressure increases and the head begins to enlarge. The neurosurgeons place tubing from the cavity in the brain to the atrium of the heart to allow the extra fluid to flow out of the brain, through the tube and into the circulation. It amazes me that something so mechanical can be placed in a human and actually function.

Even though we make six A.M. rounds, I begin to enjoy making them with Dr. Carter, the head of the department of neurosurgery. To me, he is the epitome of a neurosurgeon. He is as big as a horse with a voice twice as gruff. Everything is either black or white with no in-betweens, and he doesn't mind calling the shots exactly as he sees them. Very few people ever argue with him; none twice. He is so authoritative that if on Monday morning rounds, he tells you it is Tuesday instead of Monday, all that comes to mind is to wonder what happened to make Monday go by so fast.

This morning, we walk into a four-bed ward with Dr. Carter in the lead. He goes over to a female patient and finds she has just finished using the bedpan. He takes the pan from her and turns to one of the aides who is picking up the wastebaskets in the room.

"Here, take this bedpan," he instructs the aide who doesn't even slow down.

"No sir, that's not my job."

If there were ever a wrong time and place for that statement to be made—this was it. To begin with, Dr. Carter is "down" on the workers in the hospital. He wants to fire the whole lot, stating they never do anything unless they are told, and even then they put up an argument.

"What *is* your job?" he snaps back.

"I clean the floor."

With that, Dr. Carter turns the bedpan upside down, emptying a bedpan full of urine all over the floor. "Well, get a mop and clean the floor." He throws the pan right in the middle of the puddle and continues making rounds as if nothing has happened. No one dares laugh. Dr. Carter didn't do that to be funny. He did it to get the job done.

Two and a half weeks go by. I think I am going to make it through the month although I have slept less than any time I can remember in my entire life.

Although I can find numerous hardships to complain about, Bill Martin, the resident over me is the one for whom I feel sorry. Bill is a general surgery resident rotating on neurosurgery. He has been on the rotation for a month and is in the midst of four consecutive nights of no sleep due to a series of automobile accidents resulting in multiple head traumas. Bill is stocky, cuts his hair fairly short, doesn't give anyone any trouble, and is a hard worker. He isn't as well organized as he needs to be on this service but gets the work done, making his performance acceptable even to the neurosurgery department.

We finish morning rounds together and walk into the operating room. Barely able to keep his eyes open, he stops and tugs at my sleeve. "The thought keeps running through my mind to ask permission to go to bed rather than scrub in this craniotomy. After all, Dr. Carter is doing the case, and you are going to scrub with him; he really doesn't need any more assistance than that. Do you think I ought to ask a few hours off and get some sleep?"

I don't know why he is asking me. I certainly wouldn't want to ask Dr. Carter any favors, although I did get four hours sleep last night. "Sure, you need the sleep," I say encouragingly. We walk into the O.R. as Dr. Carter is placing the drapes over the patient.

"You going to scrub, Bill?" Dr. Carter asks without slowing down at his draping.

He realizes Bill needs sleep and if he had wanted him to go to bed, he wouldn't have asked him to scrub. From Bill's complaining, I know he doesn't think he can make it through a long operation where the skull is opened. He almost fell asleep yesterday at the operating table and kept shifting around to stay awake. I, for one, don't see how he can possibly scrub on this case.

"Yes sir, I'll go scrub," he replies.

The patient is placed in almost a sitting position with the back of the head resting in a brace attached to the table in order to keep the head motionless during the procedure. The entire body is draped in a sterile sheet and the operation is already underway when Bill finishes scrubbing and gowning. I step up to the head of the table while Bill quietly takes a position at the side of the table adjacent to the patient's lap. The circulating nurse slides a stool behind him and Bill thankfully half sits and half stands. Dr. Carter ignores him and continues to work on the scalp. Not more than three minutes pass when I hear the scrub nurse scream, "Don't! Don't!"

It is too late. Bill makes a little movement forward, then gradually leans over until he is gently lying face down on the patient's lap. There he stays. He is so still it is as if he has chosen this spot for his final resting place and is content with his awkward position of half sitting and half lying.

The nurse remains excited at Bill's act of falling asleep at the table. "Now we will have to stop the operation and redrape! He didn't have to fall on the table! How can we move him and redrape without contaminating the wound?" On and on she goes in her own flustered manner until Dr. Carter interrupts in his usual authoritative tone.

"Cover him up." He continues working his way through the skull with a drill.

"Aren't you going to move him and redrape?" The nurse asks, almost in disbelief of what she has been instructed to do.

"Cover him up with a drape."

"He will smother!"

"If you don't put a drape over him and get up here at the head of the table to help me, I'm going to get another nurse in here who will."

Dr. Carter has not disrupted his technique in the procedure one iota and proceeds as if this sort of thing happens daily around him.

There Bill lies. The nurse covers him with a sterile sheet and the team resumes work at the head of the table, ignoring the curious spectators that begin to accumulate at the door of the room, as well as the big "lump" toward the front of the table. All that can be seen are Bill's legs from his knees down with his feet firmly on the floor.

Dr. Carter wakes Bill after the case and sends him to the on-call room to catch a few hours sleep. "How can you ever expect to get a recommendation from me if you keep going to sleep on the job." Dr. Carter speaks to Bill without looking up from writing the post-op orders on the patient's chart.

Bill remains expressionless for a moment, then heads for the on-call room.

But as I watch him leave, I begin to let little thoughts enter my mind that I never before thought possible. For the first time since starting internship, a small trickle of doubt seeps forward into my conscious mind. Doubt that this system is a correct one, for the first time, doubt that my superiors are correct in their judgment of how much interns and residents can endure.

As quickly as the thoughts come, they leave. I return to my work with the compulsiveness I have learned to develop in four short months.

I continue to work: My major goal is still to become a surgeon. My intermediate goal is to become a surgical resident under Dr. Eler, and I pursue that goal with all I know to do. The immediate action goals become numerous. It is a daily battle to get through this rotation. I have to dig deep in the goal's book to keep everything in proper perspective.

Halfway through the fifth month, I am told the staff is meeting to choose the residents for next year. There are sixteen interns eligible for eight first year resident positions. I earnestly believe I am as good as the best of the interns, but what *I* think does not carry any weight in that staff meeting. I still have not been on Dr. Eler's service so he doesn't personally know whether I am a favorable or unfavorable intern. My one ace in the hole is Dr. Bowen, chief of orthopedics. I had a good month with him, and if there is a question of my being accepted for residency, I think he will stick up for me.

After the meeting, we are informed that Dr. Eler will contact us individually tomorrow.

I spot Dr. Bowen leaving the hospital and make my way to meet him just outside the front entrance.

"Could I speak with you a minute, Dr. Bowen?" I catch up and stride along with him on his way to the parking lot. He doesn't slow down.

"If you are here trying to get me to tell you whether you were accepted into the residency program, you are wasting your time. You will get the news tomorrow from the boss himself."

He won't tell me. I shouldn't put him on a spot like this.

"I had better go back in and finish my scut work. See you tomorrow, Dr. Bowen." Dejectedly I slow my pace and turn toward the side entrance of the hospital.

"Say!" Dr. Bowen calls to me after an eternity of three seconds. "Congratulations."

I turn back toward him but do not get to reply; he has already resumed his half-walk, half-run pace toward the parking lot.

I made it! I hurry back to the hospital entrance. I could work a week without sleep or food, so much adrenalin is flowing through my body. Exuberance is the feeling, knowing I got the nod to stay on as a resident. I will hurry and finish my scut work so I can tell Harriet the news.

Immediate action goals all paid off. Intermediate goal of being accepted to the residency program is accomplished. Now all that stands between me and the major goal is a multitude of immediate actions. I am finally on the last leg. The end is in sight at last.

The next day, Dr. Eler makes my acceptance into his residency program official, calling me into his office and telling me face to face. It is a good feeling, especially since I am about ready to start work, still as an intern, on his service. I still have seven months to go as an intern but will be working with the boss.

General Surgery is divided into services made up of two separate teams called the "gray service" and the "blue service." Dr. Eler heads the gray team while Dr. Jeter heads the blue team. Each team has its own chief resident, first year resident, and two interns. I am on the gray team with Paul Throm as the other intern. He has a son born a month before mine, so we have lots to talk and brag about that the other interns don't understand. Paul is a very determined worker and doesn't mind staying at the hospital on his nights off until the scut work is done. I repay his kindness by doing the same. The result is less time at home on our nights off but more sleep at the hospital on our nights on.

"Dr. Eler is going to help me do my hernia case tomorrow," Paul comes rushing up to tell me on the fifth day we are on the service. Dr. Eler tries to scrub with the interns on their first operation on his service, and it usually turns out to be an experience never forgotten; I am not sure whether he tries to make it that way or if it just always turns out to be so. Paul spends the rest of the afternoon going over the anatomy of the inguinal region, the area just above the groin where the hernia occurs, until he is sure of every detail of the operation. He has reviewed the procedure in the *Surgical Atlas* numerous times and has done several hernias at the V.A. hospital, but that isn't quite the same as doing the operation with Dr. Eler.

The following morning, Paul enters the operating room at seven-fifteen, a quarter of an hour sooner than Dr. Eler requires the interns to be there, but Paul does not want to chance anything going wrong on this case. I, along with several other interns, who have come to "watch the show," appear around seven forty-five. Paul is already scrubbed and is "prepping" the patient, washing the inguinal area for a ten minute period.

"Looks like you're about ready for the big one, Paul," I say with a grin.

"I'm as ready as I'll ever be. Look, you all don't *have* to hang around for my benefit. I'm sure I can do just as well without you." Paul is nervous but covers it up with his subtle joking.

Five minutes to eight. Paul is getting gowned and gloved and plans to have all the drapes on the patient when Dr. Eler walks in. We know he will come bounding through the O.R. doors right at eight o'clock and expect everything to be in order and ready to go. Paul has done a superb job of getting the patient ready for surgery before that crucial moment of eight o'clock.

Dr. Eler walks in, looks at our small group of interns, looks around the room and then at Paul standing in all his splendor. "Where is this patient's chest x-ray?"

Paul's shoulders drop. He knows how the boss feels about having an x-ray on the view box in the operating room. We all know it, but no one thought about it until just now; and now, everyone is ready to kick himself for not thinking of it earlier. We remember the story told to us so many times about the patient who had his hernia operated on and at the same time had a small cancer of the lung which could be seen on the chest x-ray. But no one looked at the x-ray prior to the surgery, and three months later the patient was readmitted to the hospital—dying of that cancer. I do not know if the story is true, but it is passed around as coming from Dr. Eler. True or false, it makes a point for always looking at the x-ray prior to operating, and the only way Dr. Eler can be certain we have looked at the film is to have it showing on the x-ray view box in the operating room.

To "explain" why the x-ray isn't there is an impossibility. The truth is the way out for Paul.

"I forgot to put it up, sir."

"Out."

"Do you want me to get the x-ray, sir?"

"I said 'OUT'!"

"But, sir . . ." Dr. Eler walks to the scrub sink and begins scrubbing his hands. Paul takes off his gown, removes his gloves and walks out of the room. The rest of us follow.

Dr. Eler performs the hernia operation—by himself.

That incident is severe punishment for the crime. I wonder what drives Dr. Eler to do something like that to Paul. It has upset me almost as much as Paul; that could just as easily have been me. I go to the on-call room and take time to insert some "fact" cards into the computer. I have developed a mental picture of my mind as resembling a computer. Actually, that is the way the mind works if we let it. Facts are fed in and through a process called "thinking," a conclusion is reached, the sequence being called a "thought process." I have become almost obsessed with this idea that the mind is just one big computer and catch myself using it as such. Reasoning in such a way, emotions are exempt.

The fact cards read, with no emotions:

1. There were several interns present in the operating room to watch Paul and Dr. Eler do the operation.

2. Dr. Eler has previously expressed his views on the necessity of looking at the chest x-rays prior to every operation.

3. Dr. Eler has previously instructed all interns and residents to put the film on the view box so there would be no doubt that the film had been looked at.

4. Paul had not put up the x-ray, and that act was in direct defiance of Dr. Eler's instructions.

Conclusion card:

In Dr. Eler's world, Paul was either correct or incorrect. In this instance, Paul was incorrect, so he did not get to continue with the game since he broke the rules.

According to my computer, I cannot become upset at Dr. Eler for throwing Paul out of the operating room. It was Paul's fault. Whether I would have done the same had I been in Dr. Eler's shoes is not even to be considered. Each of us has asked to be in his program and, accordingly, has agreed to play by his rules.

The incident is as easily explained as that. He is both the rule maker and the referee and all we have to do is follow the rules. I am sure of one thing: No one in our group will ever start another case without the pertinent x-ray on the view box.

* * *

The weeks pass rapidly. I do more and more operating, but the work is time consuming. I am never home and am getting to the point that little thoughts about looking for an easier place to train begin to play around in my mind. I was up all last night and will have to stay late again tonight to help out. This is my "night off," but it's too late to bother going home. I drag myself to the sleeping room. I am alone, my two roommates must still be working on the floor. I sit on the edge of the bed without turning on the lights. I'm not sure it is worth it. I am officially on call tomorrow night . . . the third consecutive night away from home. They don't have to work this hard at other places I know, and they put out good surgeons from those programs. No one can derive enjoyment from pushing his body beyond the physiological breaking point of competence; yet, it becomes a necessary evil built into a surgical program like this. Maybe I ought to go back to my old med school and finish surgical training. The night call is only every third night. However, I do not get to operate as much there.

Confusing and conflicting thoughts run through my mind as I sit on the side of the bed staring at the motionless dark of the room, not knowing whether I can physically keep up this pace for several more years. For the first time in my life I am faced with a decision of desire. My intermediate goal has been reached; I have been accepted as a resident in Dr. Eler's surgical program. I am now confronted with the truth of the matter. Do I desire to stick it out here, confront numerous immediate action goals and forfeit almost all free time, or apply to another program where life may be a little easier and with certainly more time left to spend with my young family. Comes the final day at the end of the training, I will become a surgeon, no matter where I train. Harriet has gone through so much, has given up so many of the things we used to talk about having and doing; it is almost unfair to ask her to continue through years of what the last few months have been like.

I lie back on the bed, cannot continue to let these thoughts infect my mind. I must make a decision. If I am to stay, I must remove all thoughts of leaving and never let them reappear. If I am to leave, I must begin writing applications for a surgery residency elsewhere.

I think back to the rule I made sitting at my desk the day before starting medical school—whenever a *positive* decision is made, never consider changing it; whenever a *negative* decision is reached, reconsider it after a full night's sleep. Right now, the negative is creeping in.

My decisions prior to this have been simple; list all the facts in my computer mind and almost as soon as I do, the answer comes forth. This decision is different. The facts point away from my being here in the first place, much less staying. Why would I pick such an internship to start with? The room grows darker and quieter and my mind begins to dull. The computer quits working. The power of concentration weakens until I give up any resemblance of decision-making and drift off to sleep.

I wake in the morning, quickly rehash the thoughts from last night, and come to a conclusion. I will stay here in this surgical program if Dr. Eler will keep me. I will never consider changing it. That is all there is to that.

I will protect that decision very simply: whenever a thought about leaving enters my mind, I will immediately deliver it a knock-out punch and replace it with a good positive thought about staying. I will knock out the negative thought and replace it with a positive thought. That will be the secret of controlling the situation of my mind. Once again, I add to the *Goal's Rule Book*: CONTROL MY MIND: Replace negative thoughts with positive thoughts.

Over the remaining days of internship, I come to realize the power of controlling one's mind and thoughts. After reaching the decision to remain here in Dr. Eler's program, the thoughts of leaving have never again become a problem to cope with. The remaining two months are spent maturing as an intern, readying myself for residency. July 1 makes me officially a "resident in surgery." I compare my life this past year with a patient who underwent major surgery, had post-operative complication upon complication. There were many times when the patient almost didn't survive, were times when his family thought he was not ever going to make it back home, and even at one point, the patient himself almost gave up hope of recovery. But now, he is eating a regular diet, is up walking around the room, smiles occasionally, the drains are out, the wounds are healed, and he is recovering nicely. He still has a long way to go for complete recovery, but at least he knows he is going to stick with it and walk out of the hospital a healthy man.

Two weeks ago I successfully took charge of a Code 500. It has taken me a year to fill in the divergent paths with knowledge, but I have met the challenge. I have successfully taken care of the sickest of all patients, one who was minutes away from dying of a cardiac arrest.

I also have learned a lot about the achievement of the goals in my life. I study back over my goal's book and find the rules are actually working. I am still sticking to the major goal and am still considering myself successful. As long as I continue working toward my major goal, I am a success.

I see new interns coming on service and remember back to my first day with all the uncertainties. If they will only persist for one year; if they will only persist for one day; if they will only persist for one more operation, one stitch at a time will prove them successful.

Harriet and I reminisce about the year we have just completed.

Internship was supposed to have been the worst year of the surgical program. I reassure Harriet as I have so many times in the past that our lives together are going to get better.

"I hope you are right," Harriet says. "But as long as Dr. Eler is around I can assure you, you are going to be busy." She knows too well the facts of the game called "surgical residency." She knows that the rotations are the same as in internship, but with more responsibility. She knows that she won't see much of me for the next few years. She knows too well. She won't even play the game of "it will be better" with me. All I know to do is to keep trying.

But what can insure our marriage? The divorce rate among residents is way over fifty percent. I read something in a magazine concerning this very situation: "While divorce rate is soaring, there is a solution to the problem. Statistics show that in the homes where there is Bible reading and prayer and where families go to church together every week, there is only one divorce in four hundred marriages." Now that is not bad marriage insurance. I think I will take that policy out even though I know there will be no way we can possibly attend church the every other Sunday that I am on call. Harriet agrees that it is worth trying.

So, our young family begins the surgical residency program with at least a plan. "It's going to get better. Just wait and see," I assure Harriet as I leave for the hospital for that exciting first day as an honest-to-goodness surgical resident.

Part III

GENERAL SURGERY JUNIOR RESIDENCY

I FEEL CONFIDENT, after a year as an intern, and start this year with as positive an attitude as I started my first day of internship. I glance over the new schedule telling where I will be assigned this year, and I discover that most of the rotations the first year of residency are going to be on the subspecialities: pediatric surgery, orthopedics, cardio-thoracic, neurosurgery, and urology. I had hoped to get most of the year in general surgery, rather than the sub-specialities, but guess it will be good to go ahead and get these services out of the way. If I don't do them this year, I will have to give up general in order to do them next year.

Most of my new rotations will be similar to the ones I had as an intern but the difference will be that I now rotate as a resident, not a lowly intern. I will gain experience as the responsibilities increase. The necessary scut work will be done by an intern under me. I will get much more sleep at night, only having to be up with emergency operations or complicated post-operative patients. This becomes a reward only because once it was worse. To most people, life as a resident would be so undesirable they would question the worth of going through something so terrible. I have the advantage of having lived a year as an intern, and am able to lengthen my gauge, which spans the scale from easy to difficult living; it is all relative. I would not want to go through internship again, but my enjoyment and appreciation of the little things in life have been enhanced tremendously. I will never be able to sit down for an hour and do nothing but watch whatever happens to come on television, but I will be able to enjoy time I can call my own. I will be grateful for any one hour period when I'm allowed to do anything I want, whether it is reading, study-ing, cutting the grass or sitting at home and talking with Harriet. It has been difficult to live with my entire life's saving of time stolen by the surgery department, but it has taught me something far more im-portant than how to change dressings on an infected wound, or how to restart an I.V. in the middle of the night—I have learned the true value of time. Not weeks and days, but hours and minutes and even seconds. I have learned that seconds are wasted waiting for an elevator, seconds are wasted at the operating table hundreds of times during a single procedure, that seconds have a unique way of adding up to minutes, and sixty minutes a day may be the deciding factor between a good intern and a poor intern.

I take these hard earned trophies and begin my first rotation as a resident in pediatric surgery. I begin a new page in the *Goal's Rule Book*. The anatomy of the goal structure has been easy to dissect after so many years of goal setting. I quickly jot down:

MAJOR GOAL: Complete general surgery and become a surgeon.
INTERMEDIATE GOAL: Complete pediatric surgery rotation
IMMEDIATE ACTION GOAL: See what pediatric cases are scheduled and begin reading about them—RIGHT NOW!

I have one intern under me. Only a year ago, I was the intern on pediatric surgery scrambling to get to do half the hernias and appendectomies. My policy is going to be different; hernias and appendectomies belong to the intern. I will help him on every case, but he will be the first surgeon. I will get to do some chest cases while on this rotation and will spend most of my time studying and reading about the chest related problems of the pediatric age group. I occasionally think about continuing training after general surgery and doing a residency in chest surgery. That is several years away; I don't need to make a decision now but can devote some study to it and see how much interest it holds for me.

In one month's time I perform several bronchoscopies and open two chests. Today I admit one of the cutest four-year-old girls I have ever seen. Her problem is serious; she has a completely destroyed left lung due to tuberculosis. I am scheduled to remove this worthless lung.

Dr. Bell, the chief of the cardio-thoracic department is going to assist me in the procedure. We meet at six for evening rounds.

"Do you know," Dr. Bell says as he places her x-rays on the view box, "who the patient is?"

"Rhonda Thornton is her name. Other than that I don't know what you are getting at."

"Have you talked with her parents?"

"No sir, there hasn't been anyone here with her."

"Do you mean to say you are going to take out a four-year-old girl's lung and not even discuss the operation with her parents?"

"I always talk with the parents before surgery, but I didn't see anybody with her. I'll check back later tonight."

"She is an orphan is why her parents aren't here," Dr. Bell informs me. "She is going to be adopted by Jim Teller, one of the senior medical students. He and his wife will probably be coming around sometime tonight to see her; they know you are going to be performing the operation, so go ahead and explain what you are going to do. I've talked to them once about it, but you may as well give them your two cent's worth."

I get the message Dr. Bell is giving me. If I am to be doing the surgery, I must also learn to talk to the parents. The fact that Jim is adopting her will make it that much more difficult since he knows I am a resident and have very little experience in chest work; however, this is part of the learning experience. I will tell them what I plan to do, and hope it is the same Dr. Bell told them earlier.

I begin the case, listed as first surgeon, but it is Dr. Bell who shows me where to cut, what to tie, when to slow down, when it is safe to speed up. There is no possible way I could complete this operation without his standing on the other side of the table "leading me by the hand." He explores the chest cavity thoroughly then asks me to put my hands in and feel around; shows me where to start my dissection on the lung; where to use scissors, where to use a blunt "pusher"; "assists" me throughout the entire procedure, even to the point of placing some of the closing skin sutures.

As we finish, the circulating nurse asks, "Dr. Bell, who do I list as first surgeon?"

He nods my way, "There is your first surgeon. I only assisted him."

I note a hint of sarcasm in the nurse's question but that's O.K.; I just did my first pneumonectomy whether she realizes it or not, and before I finish here, I will be doing so many pneumonectomies she won't have to ask who the first surgeon is; she will know without a doubt. One stitch at a time, I remind myself. I'll be doing radical pneumonectomies one day, but today's stitch is good enough for now; I know it will come.

Rhonda does fine. A week post-op she is running around as if she has never been operated on. She is happy when I tell her she can go home today. Looking at her jumping sparkling eyes, I can only imagine the excitement and happiness that awaits her six weeks from now—when Jim goes to the orphanage to take her home for real.

I continue to learn different surgical procedures, a whole new realm of surgery. There are many things that happen to infants and children that we don't see in the adults.

One such case is Jimmie Turner, a nine-year-old boy who hasn't had a normal bowel movement since he can remember. Each time he defecates, his rectum actually turns inside out and protrudes to the outside six to eight inches. Everytime he uses the bathroom, he has to manually push his bowel back inside. In spite of this handicap, he appears to be normal psychologically.

"I sure hope you can help me, doctor," Jimmy says sincerely. "The worst time is at school when I have to take so long to go to the bathroom." He is mature in his discussion about his problem, accepting it as just that—a problem but not a stumbling block. He and his mother live alone, and by the way they dress and talk, I assume he has had problems growing up which make his physical condition seem minor.

I assure him I will try my best to make him "good as new" within the next few days, as his eyes relate the excitement of even a possibility of being able to alleviate the situation.

I do a suspension type operation in which the colon is actually suspended from above after it has been pulled back inside as far as possible. He does well post-op and is discharged in a week. Since I first entered surgery, I have not had a more grateful patient, adult or child.

The rotation passes too quickly, like anything else you enjoy doing. On my last night as resident on pediatric surgery, I go to the resident's office to make a list of cases I performed while on the service. I do this at the end of each rotation since I will need to know the diagnosis, operation, and outcome of the procedures when I apply for my surgical board's examination. I try to keep track of them as I go along so I won't have to do all this book work at the end of residency.

I hate to see this rotation end and dread starting cardiac-thoracic surgery, as it is supposed to be the most time consuming rotation. I made it through my internship year. I will just have to buckle down and stick with it through "C-T" They do three to four scheduled open-heart cases a week plus any emergency hearts that come along, which are the worst operations because these patients usually are in very poor condition. They seldom come off the heart-lung machine without several trials, all of which means more time on the operating table. Then, with the best of post-operative care, the heart may continue to pump poorly for a few days and quit.

Lung cases are done on Mondays and Fridays. Wednesday is reserved as a clinic day to see pre- and post-operative patients. Looking over this calendar of events, I see that Wednesday afternoons are free. It can't be all that bad if we have an afternoon off to catch up on ward work, I gleefully reason to myself, only to find that Wednesday afternoons have turned into the time reserved for implanting cardiac pacemakers—sometimes very time consuming.

My primary job is to make certain the post-operative heart patients get proper care. I watch these patients more closely than on any other service since minor changes in a heart patient can mean death. There are all types of gadgets, wires, tubes, and monitors to help keep a close eye on these patients. Three small polyethylene tubes are placed in the heart at the end of a surgical procedure and brought out through the skin and connected to a monitor. One tube measures the right atrial pressure, one the pulmonary artery pressure, and one, the left ventricular pressure. Three wires connected to the chest wall transmit a continual cardiogram to a small T.V.-like screen. The first night, the endotracheal tube is usually left in place, and the patient is breathed by a respirator which has to be regulated to breathe in just the right amount of oxygen and to blow off just the right amount of carbon dioxide. This necessitates drawing "blood gases" on the patient to determine at what level these gases are circulating.

Two larger tubes, about the size of a small garden hose, are brought out the side of the chest to drain any blood that may accumulate. The blood is drained into bottles which must be closely watched to check the amount of blood loss. Yet another tube is placed into the bladder to measure the urine produced and an hourly check is made of the amount.

I only vaguely remember how to keep check on all the necessary statistics from my month as an intern. The chief resident above me will certainly help get me organized to alleviate having to rely on him for each detail.

The pediatric intensive care unit is not as well equipped with cardiac monitors as adult intensive care. The small portable units being used frequently malfunction. These monitors, metal tubes about the size and shape of a long oatmeal box with a screen on one end, connect to wires coming from the patient. The electrocardiogram shows on the screen as a continuous recording. Joe, our chief resident, sent a non-working monitor back to central supply with a note attached to have it repaired. One week later, the same monitor appears and after connecting it to a patient, it becomes apparent it was not sent out for repairs. Joe is certain it is the same monitor but to make sure it doesn't happen again he takes a 16 gauge needle and scratches a big "X" across the back of the metal plate branding it as the bad monitor and returns it with an ugly note explaining he has more to do than continue to waste time connecting monitors that don't work to patients who are just returning from heart surgery.

Two weeks later we perform an emergency operation during the night on a pediatric cardiac patient. The patient is doing poorly after surgery. We take him to the pediatric intensive care unit and hook up the cardiac monitor—it doesn't work! Joe jerks the monitor around and looks at the back metal plate; a big "X" stares us in the face. It is three A.M., and Joe is in no mood to rewrite the note to central supply explaining how stupid they are; that he is the only one staying up all night with the patients; that the least they can do is have the monitors repaired, so . . . he raises the window. I can't believe what I am seeing. He picks up the monitor and tosses it four stories to the ground. He orders another from central supply.

Word travels fast and by seven A.M., Joe is fired. Dr. Eler tells him the monitor was donated to pediatric intensive care by some women's club, and now he will have to explain its disappearance. He has a point to make and is going to the extreme to make it.

Joe is rehired within hours by Dr. Bell. A chief resident is essential to run the C-T service and there is no one to replace Joe. The next few days are rocky. Dr. Eler doesn't think Dr. Bell has any right to hire him back, but Joe stays only out of necessity.

Two mornings later as we are making rounds Dr. Eler stops and asks Joe if he has sigmoidoscoped the patient in 701 yet. This is a patient Dr. Eler referred to the chest service but left specific instructions that he wanted the patient "scoped."

The process of doing a sigmoidoscopy entails giving the patient an enema, then placing a long metal tube with a light on the end into the rectum and passing it up the colon. The patient was admitted to our service only last night and there has been no time when we could have scoped him.

"No sir," Joe replies. "We operated until four this morning and I thought I would do it during clinic."

"Let me tell you something," Dr. Eler begins, "there is only one thing everyone has equal allotments of and that is *time*. Everyone has twenty-four hours every day to do whatever he thinks is essential. Now, some of us can do what is to be done in sixteen hours and some take twenty; I want the job done and don't care whether it takes sixteen or twenty." Dr. Eler starts down the hall and stops, "What if you get another emergency right now and have to spend the rest of the day in the operating room? Would you then put the sigmoidoscopy off until tomorrow morning, and then the next? If you don't have time to get your work done and sleep too, get your work done." Joe remains speechless as Dr. Eler storms off down the hall.

"Two hours of sleep last night; that's all I got, and now I get chewed out for getting that much. I hope that evens things out between us, but I have a feeling it's only beginning."

Joe tells the nurse to send the patient to the sigmoidoscopy room . . . NOW.

We perform many heart operations on this service, plus removing several carcinomas of the lung, but the worst of the operations is that performed for carcinomas of the esophagus. By "worst," I do not mean the technical procedure is not a good operation. What I do mean is that the overall outcome for patients who have to undergo this operation is extremely poor. If I had carcinoma of the esophagus that could be surgically removed, even though it is one of the least curable of malignancies, I would undergo the operation. One surgical procedure for the tumor is to resect the esophagus and replace it with a section of colon, sewing one end to the back of the throat in the neck and the other end to the stomach. In this way food can travel from the mouth into the colon substitute and on to the stomach for normal digestion. We have such a patient, Mr. Johnson, admitted for surgery. Joe begins resecting the esophagus in the chest and I resect the right half of the colon in preparation for "swinging" it up into the chest for the suturing. The operation goes well, but on the fourth post-operative day it becomes evident the suture line holding together the esophagus and colon in the throat is breaking down. Mr. Johnson develops signs of infection in the neck area and starts draining saliva and mucus out of the neck wound. His chances of surviving such a major complication are two—slim and none. Still, we discuss what measures to take in an attempt to save him. There is reluctance to perform more surgery at this time other than to try to divert the stream of saliva from the original operative area in the hope the site will heal; all the while, the infection worsens and he develops a rapid downhill course.

On the eighteenth post-operative day the inevitable happens. The infection creeps around the left carotid artery in his neck and "eats" its way into the wall of the vessel . . . and through the wound and "blows his carotid." By this I mean blood begins to squirt all over the bed, floor, and patient. The only person on the ward at the time is a medical student who instead of grabbing the artery with his fingers to compress the source of bleeding, runs for help. By the time any of us return with him, Mr. Johnson is dead. He has bled out lying in bed. The pool of blood has "puddled" around him and is beginning to form into a soft jell. This is a terrible sight to see, especially knowing he was aware of what was happening until the time when there was not enough blood to supply his brain.

This particular situation bothers me emotionally. I can almost feel my mind changing the computer cards around so that I will have a single card telling me I dislike treating cancer patients with such a poor chance of survival. The five-year survival for this cancer is only around five to eight percent, and what we did to him seemed like a "mighty long run for such a short slide." I find it hard to accept such a low survival on these tumors, but find it equally difficult to accept that nothing can be done. If I were given a five percent chance of living, I would go to the extremes to "cash in" on that percentage; I assume these patients must feel the same way. Nevertheless, Mr. Johnson never made it to first base.

After two months on the service, I find myself fairly proficient in taking care of the patients as well as keeping up with them. There is so much data on each, I develop a system whereby I put all important data on an index card, a single card reserved for each patient. I refamiliarize myself with Mr. Harrison, an aneurysm patient, by looking at his card just prior to making rounds with Dr. Bell. It's almost like cheating to have such an impressive record of what happened day by day on a particular patient.

Making rounds has become a system of organization. As long as all the "numbers" are collected and presented, everything runs smoothly, and Dr. Bell has extra time to teach rather than have us look up information in the chart. It is remarkable how much time can be saved when a little time is spent in organizing the patient's records.

I become an organized resident, learning how to take care of critically ill patients. Many of the rules I have written in the *Goal's Rule Book* have paid off. I am organized extremely well. Each morning I make my list of things to be done in the order of their importance. Learning the impossible operations one stitch at a time has become ordinary. I find extra minutes during the day by saving seconds. The thought of immediate action goals gets me moving *right now* to get something done. Procrastination is a word I hardly recognize. Right now, right now, right now, has become my lifestyle, and I relate it all to the intermediate goal just above the immediate action goal and to the major goal at the top of the pyramid. It is all becoming automatic; the goal structure is finally forming automatic goal oriented habits.

By the end of the rotation, I have mixed feelings about cardio-thoracic surgery. It is the ultimate in the field of surgery. The residents and staff are placing new valves in hearts, cutting out lung tumors, operating in life and death situations daily; all very exciting, but the price to pay for this training is dear. Time wise, the lifestyle of the cardio-thoracic resident is very similar to the intern; the chief resident is on call around the clock, seven days a week. I am attracted to chest surgery, but at this time cannot convince myself of the added value of the extra training. I can put the problem of deciding whether to go into C-T off for a few years because I have to complete my year as chief resident on general surgery before I can be accepted to the C-T program. I will talk with Dr. Bell sometime about the possibilities. Right now, I have to start a new rotation— orthopedics. Again, I will be rotated as a resident instead of an intern. Every now and then I thank the good Lord I am not an intern; I will never have to relive that year.

Steve Webb is the senior resident on the "bone" service. I will be working with him for the next three months. The plan is for me to cover the emergency room for orthopedics every other night and he will back me.

After one week, however, I realize I am missing out on half of the cases; the ones that come in during my night off, so I discuss the situation with Steve. I am wasting some easy "getting ahead" time with this set up.

"How about letting me take first call *every* night, and if I get anything I can't handle I'll give you a call." I don't have to stay at the hospital on orthopedic call so I will at least get home for a few hours almost every night and still do a lot of bone setting and minor orthopedic surgery, as well as scrub on the larger cases. Steve agrees and the situation works out well.

This move relates back to the "do more than is expected of you" time Melvin taught me as an intern. This is not so much related to competition with other residents as it is in getting ahead with knowledge of orthopedics. Either way, every other night will be "getting ahead time" because I will be doing more than what is expected from every other resident in the program. I have successfully learned to do more than what is expected of my job; to do more than my share of the work. The *Goal's Rule Book* is holding true to form.

Harriet is beginning to wonder if we will ever have any time together. She keeps asking me if it is really going to get better once I get through residency. Will life ever get normal again? Will I ever have any time to spend with her? Will our children ever get to know me as their father who plays ball with them and takes them places? Am I sure that surgery won't always be a thief of my time? Certain doubts in her mind begin to emerge. I know what she is saying. I know what she is thinking—she may have lost me to surgery. I can tell her differently, but she sees the mold already being formed and I am slowly being poured into it. I reassure her. I reassure myself. I must guard against falling into that mold, that trap called "surgery in place of family." Yet, I must not let up now. I have too much more to learn, too many more operations to master to back off right now.

"Someday—it will be better. You'll see. It will get better." I give Harriet all the sincere assurance I can muster.

I now must put these thoughts behind me and look toward that major goal of becoming a surgeon. I must keep my eye on the finish line until the race is won.

Another day of surgery is finished. This evening I feel dead tired. I was up all last night with little piddly things in the E.R. I make it home for a late supper but am called right back to the hospital to see a victim of an automobile accident. I call Steve and tell him we are going back to the O.R. We finish operating on the patient's arm and hand at one A.M., but there are still multiple fractures in his legs to be worked on. By the time we finish operating and casting, it is five A.M. I decide there is no future in going to bed so I go up to the resident's office for coffee. We are very giddy at this time of morning, and the fact that we are two nights without sleep seems unimportant. We make rounds, eat breakfast, and go to clinic to see follow-up post-operative patients. After an hour of unstimulating clinic work I begin to get sleepy and disinterested. I look a few hours ahead and plan to skip lunch and slip up to the on-call room to catch a few hours sleep, since I will be on call again tonight.

"Come on in here," Steve interrupts my thoughts as he motions me into one of the examining rooms. "There's an old patient of mine I want you to see." I sit down beside the patient as Steve sits in a slightly cushioned chair. I vaguely hear Steve telling me about the operation he performed on this patient two months previously.

I suddenly hear laughter in the room. "Hold it right there," a surgery resident says, as he snaps our picture. I open my eyes and see the room full of residents and interns. Steve is just opening his eyes and looks sheepishly over at me. We both had fallen asleep and left the patient sitting there; he left the room and told another resident what had happened.

The resident taking pictures explains: "He said you two were sitting there talking to him, quit making sense, and the next thing he knew, you were both slouched down in your chairs asleep. When I walked in I thought I ought to capture the scene on film. I also thought I ought to bring in as many of the house staff as I could find." Steve and I remain in our original positions as everyone throws in their jab.

"If you can't take it, admit it," one intern jokes.

"Some of us have it, others don't," another chimes in.

"Real tough. Lose a few hours' sleep and look what happens."

"Hope the picture turns out. Living proof."

I can't think of anything appropriate to say. I look at Steve, he stares back with an expressionless face. Everyone thinks it is funny except us; we don't really care whether it is funny or not. All we want is a few hours of sleep—without interruption.

We catch up on our sleep and six hours later, fall back into the routine of being a resident. It is very different rotating on a subspeciality service as a resident rather than as an intern. Back then, everything was new and different. I paced myself at one hundred percent no matter what service I was on. Now, as a resident I relate my time and surgical experience back to general surgery and to what I think will be important to me after I get in private practice. I cannot force interest in the reconstructive portion of orthopedics since I know I will never be doing this type of surgery. I can no more fake interest than a salesman can fake enthusiasm for an undesirable product he is selling. I elect to spend my time on this rotation with the more practical portion of bone setting and cast applying.

Orthopedics comes to an end for me. This moment means more than just finishing a subspeciality rotation; it marks the completion of two-thirds of my first year in residency. These rotations have provided excellent experience, but I can't help being eager to complete them so I can begin my "first love"—general surgery. I still believe that general is the most diversified field in surgery because it covers such a wide range of diseases and operations, each day presenting new situations and new challenges. I must wait for that though. I still have neurosurgery and urology to rotate through.

Neurosurgery rotation for a general surgery resident is only slightly more prestigious than an intern rotating on the same service, getting to do absolutely no surgery and still being responsible for the ward work the interns don't get around to. I think back to last year when Dr. Carter made the resident scrub when he had lost so much sleep. I simply cannot see how anyone can spend his life in the field of neurosurgery. After only two days, it is developing into the most depressing rotation I have ever encountered.

I receive a call in the afternoon about a football player we are admitting from the practice field. He supposedly has sustained a spinal cord injury and is paralyzed from his neck down. Neurosurgery is expected to make him "well" again. It is difficult to remain positive on this service, but I realize my life will be miserable if I don't control the negatives by replacing them with positives.

Robert Mills, a defensive lineman for the university, had a good freshman year last year and was trying to sew up a spot on the varsity squad during spring training. He had been warned about "spearheading" tackles before; today he neared a runner, lowered his head and rammed into the runner's abdomen in order to knock him off his feet. He made a beautiful stop but lay motionless after the play was completed. He was conscious, could blink his eyelids, could look in different directions, but could not move legs or arms.

I meet Dr. Carter, chief of neurosurgery, in the emergency room to examine Robert. He is the usual muscular college football player. He does not realize the full significance of his injury and complains of missing the rest of spring practice and the probability of losing his starting position he worked so hard for. He knows he cannot move, but speaks as if it is only temporary. All his feeling will just "come back," and he will be able to walk and run and even play ball again. "Just you wait and see," he tells the coach who accompanied him to the hospital.

We operate, hoping there will be only swelling of the spinal cord—meaning hope for Robert. Dr. Carter talks of possibly being able to decompress the area and give the cord enough room to swell without compressing itself to death.

The operation is done to no avail. There is no change in any of the numerous neurological exams we perform on Robert in the following days. Weeks and finally a month passes with all hope fading for his recovery. The team gives him the game ball of the spring encounter and all the players sign it encouragingly. His attractive girlfriend stays with him almost constantly the first week, then begins to make appearances less often. By the fourth week, she is breaking her date with Robert, "just for this weekend," she promises him. I have come to know him fairly well and begin to see the inevitable changes come, both physically and mentally. I knew it could be only a matter of time before his girlfriend realized that to continue visiting him would only lead down a blind alley. There will never be a wedding, she painfully accepts the situation. The football team stops coming by so often; seeing no change, they have their own lives to live, tests to study for, dates to plan for on Saturday. Their world gradually leaves Robert out. He cannot participate in any of the activities their lives revolve around.

He finally begins the painful acceptance of reality. I do not know when he first admits to himself he is completely paralyzed. He doesn't speak of the negative aspect of his predicament—not being able to walk, run, roll over in bed—but does stop speaking of the positive situations of his once active life. He quits asking when he will be playing ball again, quits talking about marrying the beautiful girl, although he still remembers the details of their last date before his injury, and doesn't speak of his teammates. His change of conversation isn't graduated from that of running, to trotting, to walking, to standing, to sitting, to lying flat on his back; it stops just after running. He never mentions that he is permanently useless from his neck down. I do not know how to discuss the problem with him. We were never taught what to say in this type situation. No professor ever lectured on the art of discussing the future of a college football player turned puppet. The textbooks are silent on the subject. All I can offer him are my prayers and blundered conversations.

Robert loses weight quickly. The pounds melt away; not pounds of fat, but of muscle. By the end of six weeks I cannot recognize him as the hunk of an individual who was brought to the hospital wearing a grass stained football uniform. Robert has shown only one attribute that has allowed him to come as far as he has: determination to continue a productive life. He keeps his smile and begins to talk of what he may be able to do in a wheel chair, of what he will be able to do with the little bit of shoulder muscles that are left, never speaking in terms of self-pity or regrets.

What makes an individual continue to strive for high goals in situations like this is beyond my comprehension. Some of the residents comment that Robert's injury is one accident they would not want to survive. Initially, I tended to agree with them, but after talking with Robert day after day following his tragic accident, I have to disagree that his life is worse than death. On the contrary, he seems to value what little bit of physical being he has left more than some of us value a full, healthy body. Every few nights, I catch myself playing the "assuming game" where I assume that I have that very same injury and then try to decide what my feelings would be. I am unable to cope with such games and always end the session by overthrowing the rules committee and declaring "reality." I do not have the injury; I can never know for sure my reactions unless I am actually faced with the situation.

I toy with the frayed edges of the *Goals Rule Book*. I have placed so much importance on making goals, trying to accomplish them. Now it seems almost insignificant compared to the goals and rules Robert will have to make for his broken body.

A physician is not supposed to spend much time concentrating on the emotions of his patients. He should never become so involved in this aspect of his patients, only diagnose and treat. I have heard these comments, but they are lies. I am a physician. Physicians are human. It is human to have some empathy with patients whether it remains stuck back in the "storage compartment" of the brain, only making itself known in dreams, or occasionally breaking through into the conscious portion of the mind where it is either returned to the state of oblivion or expressed outwardly.

Robert Mills is not the only depressing case on the service. Case after case of head injuries appear. Some die. Some remain only vegetables. Some survive. Brain tumors in young and old alike come, many ending in death or a state of being which would have been better to have ended in death. We help too low a percentage of patients that come to the hospital; yet, no group of doctors work harder in trying to help them than do the neurosurgeons.

I am glad time has run out for me on this service. I am scheduled to move to another subspecialty—urology. I am not glad in the sense that I disliked the service or the people on it, but in the sense I keep coming up on the losing side of patients admitted to the neurosurgery service—a bullet in the head, a smashed skull, a brain tumor. I haven't particularly enjoyed working this rotation, but it is another example of what's written in the *Goal's Rule Book*. In order to achieve a major goal, I must be willing to do what I don't particularly like to do.

As I leave the service, I know this is one field of surgery I can never enter. It takes a special, objective type of individual to be able to cope with such depressing problems, and I definitely do not fit into the category. Therefore, I make a pleasing transition from the neurosurgery rotation to urology.

Urology proves to be more relaxing and enjoyable with less complicated aspects of patient care. Dr. Delbert Webb is the chief of urology, having only recently taken over the department. He appears anxious to make a good impression on the house staff working with him. The teaching aspect of the rotation is primarily derived from following Dr. Webb in the clinic to pick up as much practical advice as possible.

"One thing you have to learn is how to communicate with these old people we get as patients." He impresses upon me the fact that there is more to being a surgeon than operating. One must learn to "know" the patients, to speak their language, and to understand their ways.

It seems every male over sixty who comes to the clinic has an enlarged prostate gland, and this, in turn, causes them to have to strain to pass their urine and further causes them to dribble at the end of voiding. As the prostate gland enlarges, it blocks the outflow tract of the bladder, resulting in the patient having to get up more and more often during the night to try to empty as much out of the bladder as possible. This is the story I hear repeatedly from the male patients, the history being all the same. I even wonder why the urologist bothers to take the history, it is so repetitious.

Today is clinic day and I follow Dr. Webb from one room to another as he examines the patients, teaching and explaining as he goes. The third patient has on overalls, felt hat still cocked on the back of his head, and as friendly a smile on his face as you would ever want to see.

"Good morning." Dr. Webb speaks first. "How are you getting along?"

"Just fine, thank you."

This type of individual knows no stranger, acts as if we were both his next door neighbors and has talked to us in the backyard an hour ago. He is friendly, but not overbearing, and sits forward in his chair with both hands on his knees, one hundred percent of his attention directed toward Dr. Webb.

"I understand you are having trouble passing your water."

The old man's smile fades as he stares at Dr. Webb with awe. "Why yes, I do have a little trouble with my water," he replies.

"You have to strain a lot to get it started?"

"I sure do, I sure do." He repeats himself and looks at Dr. Webb as if he cannot believe the questions being asked.

"You have a little dribbling when you finish?"

"Why, yes! How do you know that?" His eyes widen and a slight grin appears.

"Do you get up several times at night to go to the bathroom?"

At this question the old man slaps his knee with his farm worn hand and begins to laugh. "You're too much. How in the world do you know all that about me?" I am sure he thinks he is in the presence of a magician of the first rank.

Dr. Webb assures him that many men his age have the same symptoms and all his difficulties can be relieved by a simple operation.

"Oh no! no, no. I don't need no operation." He no longer leans forward to listen to Dr. Webb but leans back and stretches his neck a few times, looking first one place and then another. He alternates glances between Dr. Webb and me. "You see, I just brung my wife to see you about her bladder trouble. She'll be back in a minute; she just stepped out to the bathroom."

Even Dr. Webb cannot keep from laughing out loud. The incident is only a reminder of the very few females we see on urology. We continue the clinic with a fresh smile coming on our faces every time we think back of the old man.

It develops that there are two sides to the coin of urology rotation. On one side is the routine; prostate gland operations, prostate gland operations, prostate gland operations. The other side is kidney transplants. The success of this operation is increasing steadily with remarkable results. Some of the problems that arise with these patients make me wonder what it will be like in the future when more and more different organs are being transplanted. Within my lifetime I will see advances in medicine that no one today even faintly considers possible. What is going to happen when the transplant of the heart, kidney, pancreas, lungs, and liver become frequent procedures at medical centers around the world? For every transplant there has to be a donor. Will the public accept giving up organs of members of the family who are dying? Once such operations become commonplace, numerous people will be on waiting lists to receive an organ to replace their diseased one. Who will decide which of these patients will receive the next available organ? If two dying patients both need one available organ, who gets it?

With the advancement of medicine, there will also be live patients who would not survive under the medical conditions of today. Such patients will be kept alive by machines which will be substitutes for their lungs, hearts, and kidneys. Who will decide when it is time to turn off the machine of a patient whose brain is non-functioning but who is "alive" thanks to the workings of the computer operated miracle machines. I am not sure. Will such patients be used as donor banks to supply organs for other patients? When someone dies, will all the organs be removed and perfused with oxygen to keep them functioning until a patient needs them? The whole business of donor-recipient can conceivably develop into a major medical and moral problem. I develop a sense of security knowing I am working in medicine of today rather than fifty years from now. The problem related to "simple" kidney transplants I am learning on this rotation are minor relative to what is in store for the future.

The routine of urology rotation continues. Surgery continues, and occasionally, death intervenes. We learn from some deaths and question others. Death is something the residents never like to discuss; but every Saturday morning, we know one thing is certain—Dr. Eler will be asking, "Why did the patient die."

Urology rotation ends. Dr. Webb gives me the usual routine about coming back to his service any time I can and spending more time with him. I have enjoyed the work, but time has come for me to put behind all the subspecialties of surgery and devote my remaining time to general surgery—my reason for being here.

I actually have a whole night off between the urology rotation and the beginning of general surgery rotation. Harriet and I have time to have dinner together and relax without having to worry about being called back to the hospital.

"Don't you think its about time we had another one?" I tilt my head and look in Harriet's eyes, waiting through a long pause for her response. I can almost see her mind working—another what?

Then it registers. She leans forward on the sofa and looks directly back into my eyes. "Another what?"

She knows, I know, and we both agree that our family ought to grow some more. Beginning general surgery rotations and beginning a larger family. How much more exciting can life get?

The weeks of general turn into months and I repeatedly am scrubbing on new operations which I have not yet been allowed to perform. I decide I must come up with some rapid learner's course on how to learn the techniques of surgery if I am ever to get ahead in this game called "residency." I review the *Goal's Rule Book* as a starter. I notice many of the residents above me are lax in attitude when they are assisting in an operation, whereas the same resident is very aggressive and attentive when he is first surgeon. As residents, we are assistants approximately half the time, and therefore, half the operating time of most residents is either wasted or yields very little to the learning process.

After some quiet time by myself I reach a conclusion, recalling the practice I made as an intern learning to perform my first amputation. I wrote the procedure down on paper and performed the operation in my mind before I ever stepped up to the operating table. Why not carry it one step further? Why not look at myself as the main surgeon on every case I assist on? I can get twice the usefulness out of my surgical experience if I pretend I am first surgeon on every case I scrub on.

I begin to apply this principle. In this way, when a patient comes into the emergency room with an injury of the magnitude that places him categorically as a chief resident's case, I try to run my mind one step ahead of the chief resident, having to make quicker decisions than the chief in order to see if he makes the same decision. Instead of passively learning from the chief resident, I actively learn by treating the patient in my mind even before the chief resident treats him. I look at myself as already being the surgeon in charge, of already achieving my major goal. I decide whether to operate on a particular patient or not; decide which emergency x-rays should be ordered; make a diagnosis and a format for treating the patient; then I check my score by merely observing what the chief resident does. I can grade myself.

I take the scheme one step further. When I am posted as "first assistant" on a case, I replace the "assistant" computer card in my brain with a "first surgeon" card and prepare for the case as if I were to be the operating surgeon. This means hitting the books the night before the operation; making myself read at least two journal articles on the diseases involved, and spending however many hours it takes to memorize the step-by-step technique of the operation. I don't let my game end when I actually step up to the operating table as first assistant. No, the game only begins at that time. I have to think fast. I have to think one step ahead of the surgeon and anticipate every advancement in the procedure. It is a mentally lost point if we come to a portion of the operation and I do not know exactly what to do next before the surgeon makes his move. I begin to see myself as first surgeon, see myself as already having achieved my major goal. These thoughts become more and more significant, so that I make another entry in the *Goal's Rule Book*: Once the major goal comes within reach, begin to see yourself as already having reached the goal. Begin to live and act as if you have actually achieved the goal. Believe you have reached your goal already.

I close the book, place it back in my coat pocket. Surgery is fun, life is fun, I am happy in this field, especially when I am operating.

Not all of the time spent in surgery is spent in the operating rooms. The clinics are necessary for pre-operative work-ups. Occasionally, a real "character" appears, and I find myself leaning back in the chair, relaxing a few moments, and just listening to him talk. I meet Silas Henry for the first time in this clinic atmosphere; a brilliant example of human nature working to its utmost to avoid being seen by a physician. I am sure some people take great pride in stating that they "haven't seen a doctor in twenty years." Silas is sixty-three and has *never* seen a doctor. Even today he is here only because he brought his neighbor to see us.

There are numerous home remedies which have "worked" from time to time and many people swear by them. It is normal for a patient to try something that worked for his grandmother years ago even though there now may be an operation or medication which would cure the ill. These home treatments include everything from cures for the common cold to ulcers, but Silas's remedy for hemorrhoids proves to be the ultimate. Many have difficulty with hemorrhoids at some time—itching, bleeding, or overt pain. Occasionally, the hemorrhoids become so bad they protrude from the rectum and result in a large clump of red, inflamed tissue that is literally "as sore as a boil" to the touch. A hemorrhoid is actually just a swollen vein just inside the rectum, becoming easily abraded when straining to have a bowel movement when firm or hard feces are present; thus, the bleeding. As they become larger, they tend to be pushed through the anus while the individual is in the act of defecation. Once outside, the anus muscle clamps down in spasm and causes the hemorrhoid to clot. The body, in turn, tries to take care of it by causing an inflammatory reaction, which results in severe pain. At this point the vein either has to be opened surgically and the clot removed, or the patient has to bear the pain several days until his body can react enough to "dissolve" or "absorb" the clot.

Such was the situation with Silas Henry. He tells of a time when his rectum was almost turned inside out with protruding hemorrhoids. I sit intrigued while he explains how he cured his hemorrhoids without surgery. For over a year his hemorrhoids had been "hanging out" and bled so much he had to wear a sanitary napkin twenty-four hours a day. They were painful, but he kept a large stock of moonshine on hand which helped ease the pain, plus giving him a good excuse to stay drunk most of the time. A friend told him of a sure cure for hemorrhoids but he could never drum up enough courage to undergo the treatment, until one day the pain became so unbearable he decided to accept his friend's suggestions. He got a dish pan, a gunny sack full of raw corn cobs, a quart of turpentine, went to the middle of a field on his farm and poured the turpentine into the dishpan. He then began to rub the prolapsed hemorrhoids with the corn cobs until the hemorrhoids were the consistency of ground beef, then quickly sat down in the dish pan. Neighbors five miles down the road heard his yell but thought it was a pig caught in the fence, he tells me.

I listen in amazement and half admiration as he tells this tale. I have to believe him because it is too farfetched to make up. Anyway, he has had no more trouble with his hemorrhoids and the feat was probably worth the pain for him. He says he still stays drunk without any excuse.

I continue life as a general surgery resident spending most of my time in the operating room and on the wards taking care of the post-operative patients. Life becomes one long routine—getting to the hospital at six-thirty A.M., working all day, staying late every other night, not going home at all every other night, not letting myself think about when it will all be over and I will get out into the real world of private practice. I approach the start of my year of chief residency. I look back to the first day I began surgery training as an intern, and realize how much knowledge and skill has been accumulated in such a short span. I plan to at least double my knowledge of surgery within the next year. Much responsibility is placed on the shoulders of the chief resident. Much attention must be given to organization, and above all, twenty-four hours a day has to be devoted to surgery. What makes this twenty-four hours a day different from every other twenty-four hour period I have spent as a resident is the fact that as chief, I have more responsibility than ever before in my life.

I have just completed my training as a junior resident, have done it with pride and accomplishment. I should be as well trained as any resident in the United States getting ready to start his year as chief resident. Yet there is still a small shadow of uncertainty which keeps poking it's head from around the corner of my mind. Once I attempt to focus on it, it is gone. I feel confident I can handle the big cases expected of me, but there is a feeling of the unknown about the coming year that makes the challenge greater than ever. I pull out my *Goal's Rule Book*. The last rule I have written in it stands out: Begin to see myself as already having reached my goal.

I look further back on the list: Proceed one stitch at a time.

O.K. I will combine these two rules and make it through the chief residency year. One stitch at a time got me through internship, and I am sure it will work again.

I am about to begin a new era in my surgical training; general surgery chief residency. It is an exciting time to actually be nearing the top of the pyramid. The view is much better up here looking down on all that I have been through. Internship and junior residency look rough having already been through them. I am not sure I could do it again. No, this is something that the body and mind could only go through once.

However, there is one dark cloud in the midst of all the excitement. Harriet is still not pregnant. What is wrong? Over two years and still every month brings hope—and then disappointment. She has been pregnant once. Why can't we do it again? I carry this hidden burden with me as I make way for the big year of chief of general surgery residency.

Part IV

GENERAL SURGERY
CHIEF RESIDENCY

THE MAGIC DAY of July 1 arrives and I become a chief resident. Under me is a third year resident, a second year resident, a first year resident, and two interns. I accept the challenge. No one oversees me except the attending staff. I call my own shots, make my own decisions, and act accordingly. The staff will come to my aid if I ask them, will assist me on any of the more difficult cases; but as of today, I begin acting as a full-fledged surgeon. I have much to learn within the coming twelve months; but now, there is one big difference—I not only have the responsibility of the patients on whom I operate, but also every patient operated on by every resident and intern under me. I will have to decide which cases the junior resident is ready to perform, and which cases I will need to do myself in order to fulfill my own need for surgical experience to become a fully trained, qualified general surgeon. What price will I have to pay for this?—One year of being on call every night, one year of seeing my wife and family only at short intervals, one year to bring together all the surgical knowledge I have acquired since that first one hour lecture in the introductory course of surgery in medical school. This price must be paid to bring it all together into one workable unit called a surgeon. I have to learn to take care of the most complicated cases possible, learn to deal with the residents and interns under me, and come tumbling out at the end of the wash a proficient surgeon twelve months from now. Numerous intermediate goals will have to be met and carried out. The *Goal's Rule Book* will have to be put to the ultimate testing. In this one year it all has to be pulled together.

Up until this time in the residency program, my main concern has been learning to operate. My "bedside manners" were learned as I progressed through the ranks of intern and junior resident, but now there are new problems to face, many of which I must decide alone. What will I be like after entering private practice? Will I be in favor of abortions? What is my philosophy on euthanasia—should a

— 137 —

person ever be allowed to die? Should a surgeon ever actually do anything to end a dying patient's life? Each of these questions is to be answered by thought-provoking hours of reasoning and questioning my innermost convictions. There has never been a need for me to reason through these questions before now. I am sure my religious background will play a role in answering these questions as well as the pressure of our rapidly moving society. *Now* is the time to start formulating my thoughts on such problems. I elect to use the scientific approach to reach my conclusions. I will postulate what I think will be my ultimate answers and spend the following year either proving or disproving the postulates.

On several occasions I have discussed abortion with my fellow residents but have never really sat down and organized my thoughts on the subject. Some of the residents reason abortion should be left solely to the woman who is pregnant. Does she, or does she not, want the baby? If she wants an abortion, she should be allowed to have one by someone trained in the technique, not by someone who has no idea of the dangers and complications of an abortion. This seems straightforward and simple enough from a purely medical standpoint, but there seems to be more to it than that, more involved than the patient and the doctor. There is a third piece in the puzzle, the embryo, the unborn. Sooner or later, our discussions center around the old question of when does an embryo actually become an "individual"—the moment of conception or when he takes his first breath? Or, is it somewhere in between during those nine months the embryo is developing into a "being" that can live and function on its own?

With such reasoning, two choices emerge. If I believe life begins at conception, I cannot favor abortion. If I believe life begins at birth, I can favor an abortion. This, I will have to decide.

Another problem I have thought about during my years as junior resident is that of euthanasia. Euthanasia is something of which very few doctors would admit to being in favor. I go back to the basics in an attempt to come up with an answer to abortion and euthanasia. I spot the Hippocratic oath framed and hanging on the wall. I do not ever recall reading it carefully for any particular meaning:

> I swear by Apollo the physician, by Aesculapius, Hydeia and Panacea, and I take to witness all the gods, all the goddesses, to keep according to my ability and judgment the following Oath:

To consider dear to me as my parents him who taught me this art; to live in common with him and if necessary to share my goods with him; to look upon his children as my own brothers, and to teach them this Art, if they shall wish to learn it, with fee or stipulation; and that by precept, lecture, and every other mode of instructions, I will impart a knowledge of the art to my own sons, and those of my teachers and to disciples bound by a stipulation and oath according to the law of medicine but none others. I will follow that system of regimen which, according to my ability and judgment, I consider for the benefit of my patients, and abstain from whatever is deleterious and mischievous. I will give no deadly medicine to any one if asked, nor suggest any such counsel; and in like manner I will not give to a woman a pessary to produce abortion. With purity and with holiness I will pass my life and practice my Art. I will not cut persons laboring under the stone, but will leave this to be done by men who are practitioners of this work. Into whatever houses I enter, I will go into them for the benefit of the sick and will abstain from every voluntary act of mischief and corruption; and, further from the seduction of females or males, of free men and slaves. Whatever, in connection with my professional practice or not, in connection with it, I see or hear, in the life of men, which ought not to be spoken of abroad, I will not divulge, as reckoning that all such should be kept secret. While I continue to keep this Oath unviolated, may it be granted to me to enjoy life and the practice of the Art, respected by all men, in all times! But should I trespass and violate this Oath, may the reverse be my lot!

I look back to a portion that may give me a guideline: "I will give no deadly medicine to anyone if asked, nor suggest any such counsel; and in like manner I will not give to a woman a pessary to produce abortion."

Does this apply directly to society today? Have the modern advancements of medicine changed this ageless oath? Is it true that we may prolong life beyond what it should be? Euthanasia can be viewed from more than one angle. *Stedman's Medical Dictionary* defines euthanasia as: 1. A quite painless death. 2. The intentional putting to death by artificial means of persons with incurable or painful disease.

Should a doctor ever intentionally put a person to death who is dying of an incurable or painful disease? I know I will never actually put someone to death, no matter how bad the disease or how terrible the suffering may be. I will never practice euthanasia. I may wish it upon myself if I were the patient in such a situation, but I would not be able to perform any act that would end a life if I were the doctor in the same situation. I cannot decide on my own that a patient has an incurable disease and would be better off dead than alive. That is not for me to say.

But this reasoning isn't exactly fair either. What about one step further? What about the patient in the hospital who has had repeated operations for cancer and is at the end of the road, dying, and nothing we can do will prevent his doing so. What about negative euthanasia? What about taking this patient, seeing him dying of an incurable and painful disease, and deciding to withhold the medications and treatments that are keeping him alive. Most patient's families would agree with such practice, but there is the problem of deciding when everything possible has been done to treat the patient. Also, what exactly does a surgeon withhold to let the patient expire? Does he actually stop the respirator, quit feeding the patient through the veins, quit cleaning the lungs out and allow pneumonia to take the patient?

I become acutely aware there is much more I have to learn these next twelve months than just how to operate on difficult cases; I have to learn things that have no black nor white, only gray; things that the surgical staff cannot teach me; things I cannot get out of a book, and cannot find at the operating table. Regarding similar decisions in my medical life, I can look back at how my ideas have formulated. First, a quite clear answer appears in the mind and goes unnoticed initially, much like a small scratch on a record; but soon the click of the scratch becomes louder until I am paying more attention to the click than to the music. My ideas and reasons seem to take shape in like manner. At this point in my residency I can only hear the faint click of a scratch and must wait awhile to see what my mind formulates. For the time being, I will continue to increase the dose of narcotics for pain until natural death brings the ultimate relief.

My first act as chief resident is to call together the resident and interns under me to discuss what I expect of them. "I have only two basic rules for you to follow—a thousand lesser rules but only two basic. The most important is to call me any time, day or night, whether I am in the operating room or at home, if there is even the slightest question in your mind about a patient's condition. I don't want to hear the following morning that you thought about calling but decided to wait until I got to the hospital to tell me about it. If something goes wrong, I want to know about it RIGHT NOW.

—— 140 ——

"The second rule applies mainly to the interns. Carry pen and paper on rounds and write down what I want done on each patient. There is no way you can remember all the things we will talk about on each patient. The only way to be sure everything is covered is to write it down. Then, don't go to bed until everything written down is checked off. I will not accept *excuses*. I will accept *reasons* why something was impossible to do on a patient, but never will an excuse suffice. I will leave it up to you to figure out the difference between an excuse and a reason.

"The next is not a rule, only some advice that has worked for me. When you write your scut work list in the morning, rewrite it in the order of importance of the work to be done, and do the work in that order. That way, even the worst intern will complete the most important jobs. Plus, your time will be the most efficiently spent that is possible."

Straight from the *Goal's Rule Book*, this has to be sound advice if they will listen and act.

I have accepted the fact that I cannot run my services properly and strive for friendship with those working under me; but I hope to gain their respect as a surgeon.

Shortly after beginning "the year of the ultimate," I am performing operations I have dreamed of doing for the past three years: taking out colons, bypassing blocked arteries, resecting stomachs and most anything else in the abdominal cavity that has a diseased segment. The scheduled cases are intriguing and educational, but the emergency, the unannounced, the unexpected proves to be the real test of ability of a surgeon.

I answer a call to the emergency room to see a seventeen-year-old boy who has been shot in the stomach. Clarence Adams lies with clenched fists, fright and pain on his face as a small trickle of blood runs down his abdomen. The emergency room intern has already started on I.V., sent blood to the lab for typing and cross matching, and the nurse has called x-ray to come take emergency films.

"Where do you hurt, Clarence?" I begin my examination.

"My back, doc. I think I hit my back." He lies straight as a board, afraid any movement may renew the initial pain of that bullet entering his internal organs, a pain he has nothing to compare with.

I roll him over to look for an exit wound of the bullet, which entered his abdomen just under his right ribs. I see nothing. "The bullet is still somewhere inside you. We'll have to get an x-ray to find out where. Can you move your legs?"

"Yes."

"Can you feel me pulling the hairs on your legs?"

"Yes."

"Have you ever been operated on for anything before?"

"No."

"Any stomach problems or kidney trouble?"

"No."

"Allergic to anything?"

"I don't know. Doc, am I going to be all right? Am I hurt bad? I'm not going to die, am I?"

"You're O.K. Hold still a minute." I examine him as I talk. I place a stethoscope on his chest—lungs sound clear; I can hear his heart sounds and they seem normal enough, feel his abdomen—no distention. I am sure there will be some blood in it, but as soft and flat as it is, there can't be too much bleeding going on in there. I again place the stethoscope in my ears and hear no sound of his intestines moving around. I glance directly at the wound—no powder on the skin. He was shot from a distance. I place my hand on his groin and feel a bounding pulse in the artery. His blood pressure is good—stable for the time being.

"Let's get those films and take him to the O.R." I motion for the x-ray technician to get a move on it. I suspect he has a few holes in his bowel that will need sewing up, maybe a hole in his liver; whatever, we'll know as soon as we open him up.

Bob First, my junior resident, injects some dye into Clarence's vein to visualize the kidneys when the x-ray is taken. We will know whether they are injured before we even open his abdomen.

The operating room is on emergency status; one working O.R., one set of scrub nurses. I call the operating room and inform them I'm bringing up a patient. I am told there is another case going on and it will be at least two hours before they finish and can free the scrub nurses to do the work.

"You put the instruments in the room and call some more nurses." I find myself gripping the phone tighter as I speak to the O.R. night supervisor. "We'll do it without nurses if we have to. I can't wait two hours to find out what's going on inside a gunshot wound." I instruct the nurse, trying not to sound too overbearing. I realize from past experience that getting the patient on the table— just getting the body into the room—is half the operation time and sometimes the most important half. "I'll have him there in fifteen minutes. See what you can do for me."

Bob and I look at the developed x-ray. "Looks like it's just below his diaphragm." I quickly glance at the x-ray and notice a bullet lodged in the vertebra; it looks like a .22. Whenever a gunshot wound comes into the emergency room I have learned to look at the x-ray to see where the bullet has lodged, then make a mental note of what lies in the path of the bullet between the entrance and where it lies on x-ray. This isn't one hundred percent accurate, but it gives me an idea what to expect. Looking at this x-ray however, I cannot decide whether the bullet is lying below or above the diaphragm. This is important because if it is below the diaphragm, I can make an incision in the abdomen and not be concerned about going into the chest. Above the diaphragm it's another Pandora's box all to itself: the heart, lungs, esophagus, and the vena cava. This would require an incision extending from the abdomen on into the chest— a much larger operation.

After studying the x-ray carefully, I decide to prep both the patient's abdomen and chest in case I do have to go into the chest, I'll have him prepped and draped already. I make an initial incision in the abdomen. There's some blood but not enough to account for a bullet going through the liver. I expect to see a gaping tear in the liver and am surprised to find such a small amount of blood lying free in the abdomen. I slide my hand over the top of the liver and find it intact. Once more I put my hand over the liver and can feel the under-surface of the diaphragm just above. There is a small hole in it with something soft plugging it. The bullet must have just grazed the top of the liver, gone through the diaphragm and into the vertebra. How can anyone be so lucky to have a bullet go through his body and not even touch a vital structure. An inch lower and it would have blown a hole in his liver and two inches higher, it would have entered the heart and would have meant instant death.

As I remove my finger from the hole in the diaphragm, the entire abdomen begins to fill with blood. Evidently, I have knocked off a clot which had "plugged the dike" and allowed this boy to live long enough to get to the hospital. Within seconds, at least five pints of blood flow through the hole which I can no longer feel and do not have time to find again. The bullet has indeed gone above the diaphragm and traversed some vital structure which has the ability to bleed out this much blood so rapidly. There has to be a hole in the heart. I have never seen a patient bleed so much, so quickly. Evidently he bled initially when the bullet passed through and formed enough of a clot to plug the hole. Now, I have undone what nature did to keep this boy alive long enough to get to the operating room. He's going to die unless I can do something *right now*.

"No blood pressure at all up here!" the anesthesiologist calls out from the head of the operating table. He begins frantically pumping blood in through the I.V.s and yells for his intern to bring all the blood he can find in the blood bank.

I quickly place a lap sponge through the pool of blood, into the area of the hole in the diaphragm. I have been in positions similar to this before, no time to think what the next step should be, only reflex actions. What I do next cannot be redone nor changed. Without hesitation I must come up with the one narrow road to take immediately or the patient will be dead before I weigh out the possibility of different routes.

I take a knife and slash the chest open. A heavy pair of scissors cuts through the cartilage between the ribs and the sternum, opening his lower right chest. Almost frantically I manually spread the wound open, only to see a pool of blood in the chest. I expose his heart and find it beating ineffectively. It looks smaller than normal. I open the pericardium, the thin sac surrounding the heart, and begin massaging while looking for the site the bullet went through. The bullet must have gone through the back side of the heart because I can't find a hole on the front. I'll never get the back side of the heart exposed well enough to close a hole. I continue massaging the heart.

There's no blood coming into the heart! I squeeze and then release my grip to allow refilling but it remains empty. After a few seconds it gradually refills and I again squeeze. I am not pumping enough blood out of his heart to keep a toenail alive, much less enough to keep his brain oxygenated.

I still assume the bullet has gone through the heart, just above the diaphragm, but feeling through the pool of blood which has not completely filled his right chest, I cannot find a hole. My mind rushes for something to do. Where else could so much blood be coming from? I ask my computer mind again for an answer; no reply. I squeeze the heart again, but it is only a time-wasting measure on my part while my mind looks for a hole my eye cannot see through the pool of blood.

The inferior vena cava! That's it! The large vein which carries blood from the lower portion of the body, comes through the liver, through the diaphragm and empties the blood into the heart. There is a very short segment of the cava which lies between the diaphragm and the heart, a space no bigger than the width of my fingers.

"I've found the hole!" I shout.

"I can feel a hole in the front and a separate one in the back side. The bullet has gone through the center of the cava. There is little room to work and even less time to do it in. This boy is dying and I have to decide how to repair the holes in the big vein and keep his heart and brain alive while I do it.

"How am I going to get to the back side of the cava to sew it?" I think to myself. "It is so short, there is no way to rotate it around and sew the back hole." Time is passing. I place a vascular clamp above and below the holes in the cava. This stops the bleeding. That much I accomplish but there is no way for blood from the lower half of the body to return to the heart, I have bought very little time to work with.

"Keep pumping in the blood!" I glance at the head of the table as I again massage the heart.

"What do you think I'm doing?" the anesthesiologist snaps back. "I've pumped in eight units already but you suck it right back out." Everyone is on edge, and for the first time I begin wondering if we are going to be able to pull it off. It is getting easier to massage the heart since it fills quicker with blood from the top half of the body but I soon realize I am not gaining much time by standing here squeezing the heart. The hole is still in the cava and needs repairing before the heart can ever pump on its own. I stop the massage.

"Pott's scissors." The scrub nurse passes them quickly. I extend the hole in front of the cava as much as possible by incising the full length of the exposed vital vein, allowing me to visualize the hole in the back of the cava from the inside. Now I am able to sew the back hole quickly without removing any of the cava. I'm left with a larger front hole to close, but I can visualize and reach it much more easily than the back. I close the back side hole and begin on the front. Bob massages the heart while I work and is able to pump blood intermittently to the brain.

"Let's see if he will come back." I finish the front suture row and remove all clamps. It is now a process of massaging the heart and hoping and praying it will start pumping on its own accord. We look at the heart but it is doing absolutely nothing. It lies flaccid in my hand with not a trace of muscle activity.

"Give me the adrenalin." The nurse passes a syringe and needle and I inject the adrenalin directly into the left ventricle. The flabby, previously unresponsive heart begins to contract. It is remarkable. The heart begins to beat forcefully and the anesthesiologist reports that he can now hear a blood pressure. The heart continues to regain its strength and within a few minutes we know it is going to hold its own.

My eyes focus on the heart. "That's about as close to dead as I'd ever want to be," I say to Bob. The tension is off, we talk, a bit more relaxed about the situation. "This fellow will never know how close he came to being called 'out' by the Big Umpire—that is, if he makes it post-operatively."

After spending over an hour closing the chest and abdomen, I go to the dressing room to change out of my blood soaked scrub suit. I remove the scrub pants, and all of a sudden it becomes real to me exactly how much blood Clarence lost. The entire front of my undershorts are completely soaked with blood. I wiggle my toes in my shoes and feel my socks soaked. It feels like walking in a mud puddle. Never before have I thought about *blood* as now. I know blood is necessary to sustain life, but have thought no further than that. There has been no reason to contemplate blood. That would be like walking outside and spending an hour thinking about the air you are breathing. There is nothing to make us do that unless we are trapped in a mine and come within minutes of running out of air. Only once out of the mine and in the sunshine would we become acutely aware of the air around us.

Two things have transpired. Clarence is in the sunshine. and I have acquired a wisdom about blood that cannot be written in a textbook. I am beginning to feel the pulsations of the life of a surgeon. It is indescribable but it is pleasant.

Clarence does make it. He is discharged after seven days without even the simplest complications following surgery. I try to explain to him what happened seven days ago on the operating table but am sure he can never appreciate the full significance of the fact that he knocked on Death's door but no one answered.

One evening after only two months as chief resident, I take some time to reflect back on what residency has all been about and how it has affected my way of thinking.

It is not all work, not all play, but it is a "way." I have slowly been pulled into this "way of life" in which the loss of sleep is welcomed—if I get to operate. The loss of time from my family; the loss of free time to play golf or tennis; the loss of outside activities on which I had once placed such a high value; the loss of everything most people consider essential to happiness; all becomes insignificant in the world of surgical residency. I awake to the fact that if I am not operating, I consider my time wasted. I feel I should do all the surgery possible in order to prepare for private practice. On top of this is added the education of when not to operate. It is equally important to know when *not* to operate as it is to know when to operate. This portion of training only increases time spent at the hospital working the patient up to see if he actually needs an operation. The essence of the residency program boils down to the philosophy: "If a patient needs an operation, operate now; if he does not need an operation, don't make matters worse by operating."

As residency has progressed, I sense I have been sucked into a hole, and how far down into it I will go before realizing there is more to life, I don't know. Rick, Bill, and Robert, the interns and junior resident are all in the same hole with me. Some day I'll make the decision how deep I must go in order to become a good surgeon and then come out, but right now all I can do is get just as deep as I possibly can while I have the desire to get me there.

With these thoughts, I rationalize my whole lousy existence as chief resident. It doesn't seem sane, but I choose to live it and pay the price to become a surgeon. I find it hard to believe I am physically able to cope, but am astonished to realize what punishment the body and mind can endure and continue to function properly. Very few are the times a resident loses a day's work due to illness; and yet, he goes without sleep for two and three days at a time; many days go by when both breakfast and lunch are missed, and dinner may not come until late. Few weeks pass that he doesn't feel he has pushed his body to its breaking point and then have to stay up a few more hours.

Usually, just before the actual breaking point, an hour or two of sleep is obtained by missing a conference or grabbing a quick nap when there is a lull in the action. Sleep and food become two priceless commodities, but given a choice between thirty minutes to get something to eat and thirty minutes to lie down and sleep, the decision to sleep always wins.

I forgo philosophy for reality; time to get back to work. I force myself not to think of the time when all my residency problems will be over. I must force such thoughts out of my mind until the last day on the service or I will not be able to survive. I have learned to control my thoughts to a great extent through these years of surgical training. If a thought enters my mind which works against my major goal, I immediately knock it out and replace it with a thought that will enhance that goal. I have labeled this the "bad apple" rule in my book. I look at it like having a bushel of apples. If a bad apple shows up, I just toss it out and replace it with a good, fresh one. It is a simple way to control one's mind.

Time passes quickly, and I begin to talk with Dr. Bell, the chief of cardio-thoracic surgery. I have decided to do chest surgery when I enter private practice, not to perform open-heart operations but to operate on the lungs. This decision has been long in coming. At first it was only an occasional thought as I watched some chest surgery, but I developed a real interest in learning how to operate in the chest and within the past month the door of opportunity has cracked open just a little bit. Dr. Bell has offered me the position of resident in his program. This crack of opportunity has to be evaluated. There is no way to become a certified thoracic surgeon without taking training in both heart and chest work. I reason with Dr. Bell that I will be wasting my time learning to operate on hearts, and I do mean time because the resident who works under Dr. Bell is on call all of the time, and post-op heart cases take more time than any other type of surgical patient. Dr. Bell replies that my reasoning is ridiculous, pointing out that time spent taking care of heart patients and operating on hearts will be invaluable no matter in what field of surgery I end up.

Just before we go to sleep, I bring up this matter of going into cardio-thoracic training to Harriet.

"You said yourself it would be like internship all over again. Why would you want to punish yourself like that?" Harriet survived being an intern's wife for a year, and by the tone of her question I am not sure she wants to go through that experience again. It is not exactly like being a widow, but it leaves a similar flavor in your mouth.

"If I don't do it now, I never will. I am psychologically prepared for it now. What do you think I ought to do?"

"What do you want to do? What do you think you should do?"

"I don't know. I don't know." I stare at the interface between the floor and wall. I do know. Why am I telling her I don't know? She knows what I want to do, and she knows that I think I ought to do. Why is she asking those questions? Why are we playing this game?

"Suit you if I go ahead and sign up for the program?"

"You are the one who has to go through it."

"You do too, in a way."

"What ever you think is best, I'll go along with."

"I think I'll do it."

The matter is settled. We prepare for bed and for a new day and a new program of cardio-thoracic resident and cardio-thoracic resident's wife.

Early in the morning, I stop in Dr. Bell's office and make a verbal agreement with him. Beginning next July 1, I will enter his program as a resident on cardio-thoracic surgery. It seems I am always biting off more than I can chew, then left with the burden of chewing it. Nevertheless, I am committed.

I refer back to my *Goal's Rule Book* . . . whenever a *positive* decision is made, never consider changing it; whenever a *negative* decision is made, reconsider it after a full night's sleep.

I have made a positive decision . . . to go into cardio-thoracic surgery. I will use the bad apple rule to control this decision. If thoughts against my going into this program come up, I will throw them away and replace them with thoughts that favor going into the program. The negative thoughts had their say-so before I decided to take up the new program, and they lost. They will get no second chance.

So, at the completion of this year, I will begin a new era in my residency training—cardio-thoracic surgery. In one way, I look forward to that day because it will mean the end of general surgery training and the completion of an entire chapter in my surgical life. My major goal moves up a notch. I realize how easy I have it right now, compared to how difficult it will be once I begin C-T. Why do

I choose to follow that path? I don't know now and probably never will. Dr. Bell opened a door of opportunity; I am compelled to walk through.

For the present time, I must deal with the problems confronting me in general surgery. A twenty-nine-year-old man tries to kill himself by putting a .22 caliber pistol to his abdomen and pulling the trigger. The bullet goes through his colon and spleen, not killing him but only necessitating an operation with fairly minor consequences. I simply cannot understand why anyone would attempt suicide. I have often wondered what goes on in such a person's mind after he has tried to commit suicide and some surgeon comes along and keeps him from dying. I am certain if this case were taken to the Supreme Court, they would rule the surgeon was infringing on the patient's individual rights. Nevertheless, this never-ending game continues to be played between the suicide patient and the surgeon. *Very seldom* does the patient win unless he blows his brains out with a hollow nose, high velocity bullet.

In this particular case, the suicide patient is quite normal and rational in discussing why he shot himself. He was not trying to commit suicide but only making a point. He thought his wife was running around, so the logical thing to do was shoot himself, reasoning that would make his wife realize how he felt about it, and then she would quit going out with another man. It is all very rational—to him.

His father, mother, and two sisters have stayed in his room almost constantly since the operation. They are shocked when I mention getting a psychiatric consultation for him. His father will not allow it, alluding to the fact that both the patient's sisters have shot themselves previously and the mother tried to shoot herself on one occasion, but the gun misfired. To this particular family, shooting yourself is a normal way to handle a problem and they are not going to let me call any "head shrinker" in on the case and give them a bad name back home.

I find it difficult to believe what I have just heard. All I can think to do is explain to them that if enough of the family shoot themselves enough times, sooner or later, one of them is going to wind up dead regardless of the point he is trying to make; and what would the people back home say then? I am sure they do not believe me. After all, they have two sisters, a mother, and now a brother who all have shot themselves and every last one of them is alive, which makes me glad I am in surgery rather than psychiatry. I don't have to explain or understand such reasoning.

I discuss such problems with the students in an afternoon teaching session. "Suicide is one problem I do not understand, and alcoholism is another. Habitual drinking is a dreadful thing to contend with from both the patient's and the surgeon's viewpoint.

"I say 'habit' rather than 'disease,' because I feel it is not a disease process that a person can 'catch' or 'come down with' or discover he has. I look at it as a habit, just as smoking is a habit. Some individuals are more prone to be controlled by a habit than others, and these individuals become what is known as alcoholics." I enjoy lecturing to the students working with me. It's informal, easy talking with no quizzes.

"One of the end results of drinking is cirrhosis of the liver. It is an intriguing subject to study since it results in both a psychological and anatomical change in the body. The liver becomes scarred and loses its ability to function properly. The venous blood from the intestines and spleen normally flows through the liver and on to the heart. However, when cirrhosis develops this blood pathway through the liver is 'dammed' or blocked. Pressure builds up behind the dam and the blood has to find another route to the heart. One such route is through the veins in the esophagus. By using these veins the blood can bypass the liver and empty into other veins leading to the heart. As with any compromise by the body, a price must be paid. The only way this route will suffice is for the pressure in the veins to increase enough to 'push' the blood through the esophageal veins and around the liver. These veins in the esophagus are not accustomed to a high blood pressure, and once all the blood quits going through the liver and begins using this route as a bypass, trouble develops. The veins in the esophagus become engorged with blood, dilate, and become tortuous, giving the gross appearance of long worms wiggling their way up the esophagus. Such distended veins are called 'esophageal varicies,' similar to the varicose veins found in the legs. They are very fragile and frequently bleed, resulting in a massive amount of blood flowing into the stomach, only to be forcefully regurgitated back up the esophagus and into the mouth. Each time the patient vomits, there appears to be a quart of blood. and the patient and doctor alike think the patient will surely die.

"If you take the overall number of cirrhotics who bleed from varices, seventy percent will die within one year and sixty percent who have bled once will rebleed within a year. These numbers are fairly consistent whether the patient is operated on or not. For this reason, many internists and surgeons do not believe such a patient should be operated on since they do not feel it can increase the overall survival rate. However, there is no doubt that some of these individuals are indeed saved by the knife. Such patients are bleeding to death. Every non-surgical method of controlling the bleeding has been exhausted, and there is no hope for the patient other than surgical attempts to shunt the blood away from the esophageal veins, thus relieving the pressure in them and stopping the bleeding."

I complete the mini-lecture to the students and realize that with only two months left in my chief residency program, I still have not performed one of these shunt operations. These alcoholic patients I have consulted with either died a rapidly bleeding death, or quit bleeding and refused surgery.

Within two weeks, two patients come in for shunts. The second has just arrived in the emergency room. Her name is Jeannie Franco. When I arrive, she is in the process of vomiting huge quantities of bright red blood into a plastic blue-green basin a nurse has handed her. I am one of the first to see her and insert a long tube into her stomach. There is an outer balloon around the tube and by inflating, it will "hold pressure" against the bleeding veins temporarily. I inflate the balloon and Jeannie's bleeding stops. The situation is under control for the time being; the only problem is that the balloon cannot be left inflated indefinitely. I will leave the balloon inflated for an eight-hour trial period. At the end of that time the balloon will be deflated and the situation re-evaluated. The veins will either begin rebleeding massively or there is a chance they will not rebleed, and this will give us time to get her to surgery before the "finger in the dike" lets go again. There is no way to predict whether an individual patient will rebleed or not. We just wait the eight hours, deflate the balloon and see.

Both Jeannie and her husband are in their late forties, both alcoholics who could "never seem to stop drinking," as her husband puts it. He is about as scared as an individual can be from all this bleeding. He has blood on his shirt and pants from Jeannie's vomiting; He has assessed the situation correctly—Jeannie may die.

The time passes and the balloon is deflated. Blood fills her mouth, flows over her chin, onto her gown, starts to soak the sheets. I quickly reinflate and the faucet is turned off once again.

Jeannie looks at me with pitiful, sorrowful, eyes. It is amazing what eyes alone can relate. Her eyes repeatedly try to capture mine as I busy myself getting the tube fixed. She is afraid of dying. It is real to her. She wants help but can only beg for life with her eyes, knowing the seriousness of the situation. She is helpless, totally dependent on someone else. She keeps looking at me, never moving her eyes from mine.

The internist is present and the care of the patient is partially his. His advice has to be honored in this situation, there is no absolute answer. He asks for another twenty-four hour trial and concedes to surgical intervention if she rebleeds at that time.

Medical management is not going to work in this case. I will perform the shunt operation to relieve the pressure on the veins, and she will die post-op; the story I have heard so many times about these patients.

Twenty-four hours pass, and I alert the operating room that I will most likely be bringing a patient down for a "shunt." I check the blood bank to make sure they have set up the six units I ordered for the possible operation.

I again deflate the balloon. She bleeds massively. I reinflate and order her directly to the operating room. I take a few minutes to talk with her husband before going into surgery.

"She's in bad shape, John," I begin. "Her chances of pulling through any type of surgery, especially an operation of this magnitude, are not good. Even if she does, I will guarantee you she will be dead within a year if she doesn't completely quit drinking."

"Oh, I'll make her stop drinking," John replies in all sincerity. "I'll see to that."

"I don't believe you," I tell him. John appears hurt by my statement. "The reason is that for her to quit drinking, you have to quit."

He is angry and his voice cracks as he speaks. "I can do anything for my wife. If she lives through this, you'll see." He heads for the waiting room without waiting for a reply.

I complete the shunt operation with some difficulty, but the bleeding comes under control. There is no more bleeding after the operation and Jeannie remains in the hospital three weeks. The day finally comes when she is ready for discharge . . . alive.

"Jeannie, I hope you and John have talked things over about this drinking problem. Your liver will never be normal and you have undoubtedly cut off many good years of your life. However, you will cut them all out if you don't start taking care of yourself." My sermon over, I wonder how much good it has done. She would not understand my *Goal's Rule Book*, but she had better learn fast how to set one particular goal and make it: to quit drinking.

I see Jeannie and John at the clinic two weeks following discharge. They are all smiles and reassure me they have both quit alcohol and have not touched a drop since her operation. I express interest, but retain serious doubt their good intentions will survive. In this particular case the operation saved Jeannie Franco for the present and she has benefited both physically and mentally from her encounter with near death. Will she be a "lucky one?" Will I ever again operate on a "lucky one," or will they all fall into calculated "death numbers" the internists and surgeons discuss so much? I don't know whether I will ever know about the others, but Jeannie and John don't particularly care about them. She has beat the "numbers"—for the time being.

I make it home tonight at a decent time. For a change, Harriet and I are able to eat at the same time. I begin telling her about my discussion with the students, and about how bad a patient with cirrhosis can bleed and about Jeannie and her husband, John, and how I hope they quit drinking. As I talk and eat and talk some more, I gradually realize Harriet is not listening to me. She is acting like she is listening, but I know she isn't.

"Do you agree?" I ask her.

"Yes, I agree." She responds.

"You agree with what? You don't even know what I was talking about. There was nothing to agree with." I begin eating again.

"You want another boy or would you rather have a girl?"

"You're pregnant!? I can't believe it."

"I've already been checked."

"This is great. Boy or girl. Whatever you want to have will be just great with me."

The excitement of another child keeps me awake, just thinking about having another one after trying for so long.

The next day picks up where yesterday left off. Surgery in the morning and clinic in the afternoon.

I stop in the resident's office after completing clinic and notice a small typewritten note in my mail box. It is from Dr. Eler.

Private patient coming Sat. afternoon. Mr. James Clement. Needs E.C.G., chest film, liver studies, sigmoidoscopy on admittance. You will get above done
        YES   NO   (CIRCLE ONE)

Typical. I have come to know he doesn't like "words." He sends notes to be checked "yes" or "no." He doesn't care whether I have a good reason for not doing something; he only cares whether the job will be done. If I were going to be out of town for a meeting Saturday, I would not try to explain, I would only circle the "no" box—or cancel the trip and circle the "yes" box and be here when his patient arrives. As I analyze his system of doing things, I begin to appreciate the core of his thinking process. He doesn't know what the word "can't" means. To his way of thinking, anyone can do anything he sets his mind to. I agree; that is basically true. We all do what we want by a process of reasoning called excuses. I can be asked to do something completely within my power and come up with the correct excuses not to do it. Dr. Eler gets only the basic answer to all his written questions and requests. He does not allow for any excuses and, therefore, an honest answer is the result. Furthermore, he doesn't have to listen to all the problems of everyone under him.

I circle "Yes" and slip the note in the "out" tray on the secretary's desk. As I near the end of my chief residency on general surgery, I can look back on it with pleasure. True, it has been a rough year with many disappointments but also many rewards. I've learned that I cannot completely control what happens to every patient on whom I operate. Some develop problems and complications I cannot explain, and some I think will surely die recover for reasons I cannot explain.

I have learned to appreciate and respect *time* like no one else could ever possibly understand this precious commodity. This past year, I have had no nights off, no weekends to call my own. Anytime I have been away from the hospital, I have carried a two-way radio in order to be available since there is only one chief resident for each service and there is no one to cover for me. I remember in February when my parents came to visit for a week, I could count on one hand the hours I had been able to spend with them. I remember the occasional weekend nights Harriet and I would visit with friends, only for me to fall asleep on the sofa or be called back to the hospital. It does no good to explain to anyone what it is like being poor. I do not speak of money, but of free time. It has been like going for an entire year with no money in your pocket with no glimpse of better days. A man can work two days and nights consecutively without sleep if he knows he will be off at the end of that time. But how terrible it is to start into that second night without knowing whether it will end in a third night without sleep or in a period of respite.

The only consoling thought I keep tucked in the back of my mind is that the day will eventually come when I will finish residency. No job in the world can be this time-consuming. I am already forgetting many of the sleepless nights I have spent in the O.R. and wonder how long it will take after residency before I forget how difficult it really has been. I want to forget many of the bad times, but I think I should hold some of this putrid existence in my mind, just to have something to compare life with. As long as I keep some of this in my memory bank, I will always appreciate relaxing for five minutes without really having anything at all to do, will be able to enjoy sitting on a hillside surrounded by nature a thousand times more than anyone else. A vacation will always be a treat I will forever be thankful for; each weekend of leisure will be a million dollar treasure that can never be sold. I will never waste time unless I pre-plan it as a needed time for rest, will never watch television unless I choose to waste the time. In these short years, I have learned the true value of time, and anyone who threatens this cherished portion of life will be looked upon as a thief and an enemy. Time has become all-precious to me.

With only one week left as chief resident, I do not schedule any surgery, but plan only to assist the junior resident on any cases he would like to perform. The only case he can find for my finale is a woman with a breast lump that looks suspiciously like cancer. She noticed the lump four months ago but sought medical advice only recently. I don't understand how a woman can let something like this go unchecked. I realize there is a natural fear of malignancy, but the one thing that will ultimately bring death is a cancer which is inoperable, or unresponsive to radiation or chemotherapy. It doesn't take long for a patient to come face to face with these facts. I choose that subject as my final lecture to the students on the service.

"When one speaks of curing cancer, the average layman does not realize there is a separate cancer for every organ and every different type of tissue in the body, and numerous doctors and technicians are spending their lives trying to find cures for these different types of cancer. To speak of 'cancer' as a single entity is like lumping all the songs ever sung into one bucket and calling it 'song.' Each type of cancer is different, just as each song is different. To learn a cure for one cancer does not necessarily mean learning a cure for all cancer, any more than learning to sing a particular song means that you have learned to sing all songs. Some types are more common than others, breast cancer being the most common in women and lung cancer the most common in men. Both of these tumors are well known to the general public, and symptoms are taught in order to either prevent the cancer or find it early enough to have a chance of cure. Still, people ignore these facts on these common tumors which kill men and women by the thousands.

"A woman will feel a lump in her breast, and the first thought which comes to mind is not—'I had better go have this checked,' but 'maybe it will go away.' Worse still, most women will not even check their breasts themselves because they fear they will find a lump, and this would necessitate a decision. They are afraid to make a decision that might be life-threatening. At the other extreme are the women who come almost monthly to have their breasts checked because they keep thinking they feel a new lump. I try to tell these patients to check themselves once a month, just after their period starts; no more and no less. Then if they feel something significant, come in for a check-up. But my suggestions go unheeded by the majority.

"Once a persistent breast lump is found, most physicians recommend a biopsy. When the time comes to discuss surgery for such a lump, all reality unfolds itself to the doctor and the patient. The reason for the operation is to take out the lump to see if it is malignant or not. If it is not a malignancy, then the procedure is complete and the patient returns to her room. If it is malignant, off comes the breast, and the patient does not know the outcome until she awakens from the anesthesia. The real problem comes in the doctor's office before the patient ever comes into the hospital. No matter how much the surgeon believes the lump is not malignant, he has to explain that the patient needs to give him permission to remove her breast in case it does turn out to be cancer. At the time, all reality is made manifest. The surgeon realizes there is a chance it may be malignant or he should not ask the patient to go through the emotional strain of actually signing a piece of paper giving him permission to remove her breast. The patient herself faces this same reality that even though the surgeon has told her it is most likely not malignant, he is still requiring her to sign a statement giving permission to remove her breast. The emotions are the same whether she does or does not have breast cancer. Perhaps this is why women defer checkups on breast lumps."

As I leave the lecture room, I realize I won't be lecturing to these students again on general surgery. I have mixed feelings but mainly, it's a good feeling to be this near through.

The remainder of the week glides by easily for me. The junior residents, who will become chief residents in a few days, have already taken over; I wander on up to the cardio-thoracic section to see what is in store for the remainder of my residency. The one thing I notice immediately upon making rounds on C-T is that these patients are sick and many will die if hour by hour tabulation is not kept current. I thought time was of essence this past year, but I begin to wonder if I haven't just come off a vacation, getting ready to start work. I don't see how there is enough time in a day to do everything expected of me. However, it is the same feeling I had starting internship, junior residency and chief residency in general surgery and feel confident this will be no different. Twenty-four hours will come and go every day, I will make it through each day the same as I have done before. The *Goal's Rule Book* becoming worn, proving itself true as I begin the last mile of my goal journey . . . one stitch at a time.

My last day as chief resident on general ends without incident, no cap and gown, congratulations, nor goodbyes; just finish one aspect of training and begin another.

Part V

CARDIO-THORACIC SURGERY RESIDENCY

THIS IS AN UNUSUAL transition period for me, having completed general surgery training and starting a completely different type of surgical training program. By the end of my year as chief resident on general, I felt competent to perform any operation that came my way. I could go out into the "real world" and start practice as a general surgeon, never have to enter the chest cavity, and be completely competent in my work. However, starting today, I am again like an intern starting the first day on the surgical service. Of course, everything is in a different perspective concerning patient care: what is expected of the residents, the enormous responsibility placed on my shoulders, and a continuing development of the secret of running the residency portion of the program—organization.

Dr. Bell is my new boss. He is the one I have to answer to, and he has instructed me how to answer. If he asks a question concerning a patient, he wants one of two answers without hesitation, a direct answer or "I don't know." He taught me this in one short episode over a year ago when he asked a question related to a patient he had referred to general surgery. I hesitated only momentarily when he blurted, "You either know the answer or you don't. If you don't, just say so." Ever since, I have felt free to be perfectly honest with him in my answers, and I believe he has more respect for my answers since I conformed to his basic idea of being completely honest with each other.

Dr. Eler is past tense and although he taught me most of what I learned in general surgery, I now have to gather the knowledge of surgery of the chest from the head of the cardio-thoracic department—Dr. Bell. He has chosen me to be his number one resident. I have control over three individuals and am solely responsible to him for every action any of them makes. I am assigned one junior resident who is on call twenty-four hours a day while he is in the cardio-thoracic service. I will be the only one to tell him when he can go home, when he has to stay up all night with a patient, when he can sleep; about the only thing he will be allowed to do on his own is breathe. I have never had such responsibility before, and must learn to act fairly or lose the ever-important respect of the trainees working under me. I cannot let the junior resident pass the breaking point where he becomes so inefficient he becomes useless. I will have to share my sleep ration with him and still acquire enough sleep myself to remain physically capable of standing at the operating table for the full endurance of an open-heart procedure.

I am given two interns, each remaining on the service for a one-month period. It will be the most difficult month of their internship, and they have to accept it as that. They alternate night call and they're expected to remain at the hospital watching the post-operative patients like a new mother the first night at home with her baby. There is no on-call room for the interns on C-T—very seldom will they be allowed to sleep. There is no reason to have a room assigned that will never be used. There is no way I can be fair to them concerning the amount of sleep they will get during the one-month period on the C-T service, no way I can relieve them from some of their duties myself. I will be up at night often enough as it is and then be expected to operate hours on end the following day. They will have to survive only a month. I have to survive many months after they have rotated off C-T, so I must pace myself for the duration of the time. They will dislike me but I have no alternative. I experienced the same month when I was an intern on C-T.

These three individuals and I make up the service. I am supposed to be the most highly trained resident in the hospital and am expected to exhibit stately leadership to those under me. Yet, I make rounds the first day on the service with all the uneasiness of an intern making his first rounds. No one knows this because I keep it as an inner feeling, afraid to express it openly. Part of leading this group is based on respect for leadership, and I have to sustain that respect I earned from being their chief resident on general surgery. Nothing in the goal's book can help me here. It's a new experience.

I have proved myself in medical school, internship, and the general surgery residency. Now I have to start anew to remove the lung, to close holes in infant hearts and replace valves in adult hearts, study the arteries in the heart and know where to sew vein bypass grafts around blockages, and learn to deal with emergencies of the chest in situations where I will face the problems alone, and reason only with myself concerning what to do. In addition, I will insert cardiac pacemakers in hearts that do not beat at a normal rate. I have all this to learn in the months ahead and cannot help but feel some apprehension as I begin this final, but most difficult portion of training. I look forward to the day I can look back on surgical residency as the end of a chapter of my surgical career. Then, I will be competent. There will be no fear to hide, no apprehension to cover up, no false leadership required. But enough of that thinking. I must first live this final chapter without letting up.

I plan to enter this first month with caution. I don't want to start the year off poorly. I will be assisting Dr. Bell on the heart cases for the first few months in order to learn how to put a patient on the heart-lung machine and see how most of the operations are performed before I get to become first surgeon.

The first month proves interesting. I assist on several open-heart cases and am putting the patient "on the pump" after only two weeks. I learn to split the sternum or breastbone, and insert tubes into the veins going into the heart, connect these tubes to the heart bypass pump in order to drain all the blood going toward the heart into the pump. Another tube is passed from the pump and inserted into the aorta, the large artery coming out of the heart. In this way the heart can be completely bypassed, opened, operated on, and closed again; all the while a mechanical pump is keeping blood flowing through the body. Putting a patient on the pump is very minor relative to the actual cardiac procedure, but it is a big step in the direction of actually getting to operate on the heart. I perform this part of the operation as if it were the most important step in the procedure. To me it is. If I do not learn to do it well, I cannot expect Dr. Bell to let me move onto the actual open-heart portion of the operation. Rule book again—one stitch at a time.

I feel elated, astonished that the first ten procedures are all successful and without major complication. It is difficult to believe a human heart can actually be cut open, sewn back together, and still function in any resemblence to normal. Open-heart surgery is the biggest single advance in the field of surgery since the beginning of anesthesia. Countless people have benefited from operations which have been truly life-saving. Numerous others are able to live active and useful lives only because a heart valve can be replaced, or an abnormal opening in the heart sutured close, or a vein used to bypass a blocked artery. However, these great benefits are not obtained without a price. New techniques are being developed. New techniques are not always successful, though; no new operation can carry a guarantee of success—only of hope.

There are few "second chances" with heart surgery. Operating on a diseased heart is a game of perfection for the perfectionist. A single mistake may lead to catastrophe. A short-cut on the operating table may result in the heart never beating on its own again. A wrong decision at a critical moment in the procedure may bring death.

These facts are superfluous to me at the present. Their meaning cannot be appreciated until I am placed in the situation of actually operating on the heart. Being told these statements is like reading sentences out of a surgical manual, like reading a menu but never eating the meal. I will have to experience cases that do not turn out as expected; cases that will make an imprint on my mind in such a way I will never be able to forget them. This will be my learning. process, just as it has been through internship and general surgery residency. I can be told, but I must see; I can be taught, but I must experience. In reference to the *Goal's Rule Book*, I now need both "I have to go through myself" and "I don't have to go through myself" experiences. Right now, I dread some of the former.

I finally get to perform my first heart operation; the simplest of them but a giant step in the right direction. It is called a Mitral Valvulotomy. One of the valves in the heart is scarred as a result of rheumatic fever and has closed the opening between the two chambers of the heart to such a degree that the blood flow through it is greatly impeded. I place the patient on "bypass," open the heart and make two small incisions in the scarred valve, opening it to near original size.

The patient does well post-op, and I make ready for larger operations. There is all the difference in the world when I am first assistant on a case that I know I will be first surgeon on within a few weeks. I mentally check back into the *Goal's Rule Book*: I picture myself already having achieved my goal, picture myself actually already performing valve surgery. Even though Dr. Bell is doing it with *his* hands, I am doing it with *my* mind. As I assist him, I make numerous mental notes concerning the minute details of the case: how he holds the tissue forceps when in a critical area of the heart; how many knots are necessary for each suture when sewing in the valve; what size suture he uses; how he makes sure all the air is out of the heart when the procedure is completed. I want to be able to do it all without having to rely on him for the next step. I want to be proficient enough on the first artificial valve I put in so that I do not have to ask a single question related to the technique. I have even forfeited my secret closet of time just prior to going to sleep, and now any time I lie down during the night, I think myself to sleep by mentally going over the operation step by step. I always drop off to sleep before finishing the procedure, but know I am ready to put in a valve.

I wander into the intensive care unit, the I.C.U., before going to bed to make a last check on the patients. The unit has seven beds, supposedly split between cardio-thoracic surgery and general surgery. As I begin rounds I realize C-T has all seven beds filled with the sickest people in the hospital. I pick up a chart and sit down in the large easy chair in the corner and flip the cover of the chart open. Instead of reading the page of intern's notes before me, I only stare at the chart and reflect on the preceding week, the most difficult I have lived through. We ended up doing four hearts, a thoracic aortic aneurysm, and esophageal lye burn, which destroyed the esophagus, stomach, and first portion of the duodenum. The burn patient died, and we had to take two of the hearts back to the operating room because of rebleeding. One of the rebleeds occurred while I was operating on the esophageal burn, and I had to get someone else in to finish the case while I took the heart back to the operating room.

I continue staring at the chart. I cannot run any faster. It's been like trying to drink a waterfall. I can't handle any more. Hearts rebleeding, people swallowing lye trying to kill themselves, seven patients in I.C.U. requiring personal attention. The only thing I have going for me tonight is that there are only twenty-four hours in a day and then another day begins. I am tired and sleepy. It has to look better after a few hours of sleep.

I force myself through the check of patients in the unit and settle down to study the chart of the next patient scheduled for open-heart surgery. It looks like the most difficult case we have encountered this year. The patient is a sixty-three-year-old female who survived a heart attack several years ago but was left with an aneurysm of the heart; a ballooning out portion of the heart which robs the rest of the heart of it's efficiency. This area needs to be removed before the heart completely gives out.

I complete my work-up on Mrs. Krozier and return to the

resident's library to begin a review of aneurysms of the heart. I make myself read everything I can find about each case I scrub on, a rule I made as an intern that I still stick to. I already know in a general way what the pathology of the case is and what operation will be needed, but I must now learn the details of the disease process and operation. I must learn more than I will ever have to know about each particular operation because so much of the detail will be forgotten with time. After beginning to read about the aneurysm which is causing Mrs. Krozier's heart failure, I see that following a heart attack, the wall of the left ventricle of the heart may begin to bulge, much like an inner tube sticking out through the side of a tire. The problem this causes is not one of rupturing, but the fact that this portion of the heart is not doing its share of the work. As the aneurysm, the ballooning-out portion, enlarges, more and more blood in the heart stagnates in that area and is not pumped into the body. Mrs. Krozier is in heart failure due to the aneurysm and cannot do much more than go from her bed to the table without sheer exhaustion. The operation will be to remove this portion of the heart and let the remaining heart muscle carry on the needed pumping action.

Two days later, we make ready for the operation. Dr. Bell will perform the surgery and I will assist. We start at the usual seven A.M. operating time. Everything goes well. Dr. Bell places her on bypass and excises the ballooned out area of the left ventricle. A piece of muscle about four inches in diameter has to be removed in order to excise the aneurysm in its entirety. Looking at the heart, I can easily see why this portion of muscle is not able to pump. It is less than a quarter of an inch thick and shows no sign of activity at all. The area is cut free, leaving a large hole to be brought together by placing sutures through the remaining edges. The muscle looks and feels like soft fish flesh rather than the normal firm cardiac muscle. Every other stitch Dr. Bell places pulls out and has to be replaced but finally he places the last stitch and no leakage of blood comes through the newly placed suture row. He has done a superb job of closing the defect left after removing the aneurysm.

We take her to the recovery room and keep close watch on her for four hours. Very little blood coming through the chest tubes. She is stable. We next take her to the intensive care unit, hoping the critical period has passed and we have been able to pull her through without a major complication.

Everything is going so well with Mrs. Krozier, I take some time to explain to the medical students on our service the purpose of chest tubes following open heart surgery.

"A blood thinner is used during the operation to keep the blood from sticking to the heart-lung machine, preventing clots in the system. At the end of surgery the thinner is neutralized to a certain extent, but there is always a continuous oozing of blood for a few hours. The blood accumulates in the chest and is allowed to escape to the outside through these pliable plastic tubes placed through the chest wall and connected to the bottle on the floor. The bottle has markings which allow measurements of how much blood is lost each hour. Eighty to one hundred cubic centimeters is the upper limit per hour. If too much blood comes through the chest tubes, this indicates the bleeding inside is more than just ooze from the operative site and the patient has to be reoperated on to find and control the hemorrhage."

The students listen intently, but they will never be able to appreciate what I am saying unless they someday operate on a heart, stick in chest tubes, watch how much blood comes through, and have to make the final decision whether or not to take the patient back and open him up to find the site of bleeding. I conclude the mini-lecture and relax.

It is ten P.M. and there's not a trace of trouble. I enjoy taking care of a patient who does well after surgery. She still has an endotracheal tube in her windpipe and is connected to a respirator. Essentially all I have to do is regulate the machine to keep her breathing normally. I go over a few more of the basic mechanics of post-op care with the students and few appear interested enough to stay around past bedtime to ask questions. I dismiss all but two who will remain with Mrs. Krozier all night to observe the actual post-operative care on an open-heart patient. She is putting out about eighty c.c.'s of blood an hour, about a Coke bottle full, and I am content to accept this amount of loss through her chest tubes.

All of a sudden I notice blood pooling under my feet. My mind rushes for an explanation. I want a simple solution. This is the first time I have been confronted with a post-operative complication that I have not been able to reason out almost as soon as the problem unfolded. "There is a unit of blood running into her I.V. It must be disconnected and leaking onto the floor," I think quickly to myself.

This reasoning proves false as I glance at the I.V. tubing and find it intact. Blood is now completely covering the floor under the bed. I kneel to look for the source under the bed and see the chest tube bottle, which collects the drainage of blood coming out of the chest through the plastic chest tubes. The bottle is sitting in place on the floor at the other side of the bed. It is completely full of blood and actually spouting out the small hole in the top! I cannot imagine what is going on. All I can think of is getting her back to the operating room where we can do something about it—whatever it is. I yell at the intern to grab the chest tube bottle while I disconnect the respirator and start using the oxygen bag to breathe for her. The intensive care nurse excitedly tells me she is notifying the operating room that we are on the way with a patient.

The elevator. Why doesn't the elevator come so we can get her to the operating room? Everything is so pressing! Time is so important!

We wheel Mrs. Krozier into the operating room and I quickly open the chest. By now I realize the only thing that can cause this much blood to show so quickly through the chest tubes is a rupture in the suture line where we had such a difficult time getting them to hold together. I get the chest open and sure enough, the lower end of the sutures has pulled out of the heart muscle and blood is pouring through the opening. I grab a gauze tampon and place it over the hole to stop the bleeding, look up and see Dr. Bell making his appearance in the O.R. The intensive care unit nurse had presence of mind enough to call him at home and tell him of the problem.

"What happened?" He begins getting gowned and gloved. I have never been more glad to see anyone in the whole wide world as I am to see Dr. Bell.

"Part of the suture line tore loose in I.C.U. Blood started pouring out her chest tubes all over the floor. It scared me; I couldn't figure out what happened. It looks like about half the sutures have pulled through.

"I thought we had gotten her through but this is a mess." Dr. Bell is now at the table assessing the situation. "Nothing to do but try again."

We begin pumping blood back into her and finally start to obtain a decent blood pressure. Dr. Bell begins the tedious process of trying to place stitches into the muscle which has proven to be so fragile. He places the last suture into place and ties down. No more leaks. The drama is over. He has successfully reclosed the tear, and we must now repeat the post-operative care which we started so many hours before.

I look at my watch and see three-fifteen A.M. staring at me. I'd completely lost track of the time. All is quiet and by some miracle, Mrs. Krozier is not only alive but is stable once again. I decide to get some sleep, leaving the intern by the bed to keep a watch on things.

At four-thirty, I am awakened by the intern yelling at me to come back to the intensive care unit. I run in. There is blood all over the floor under the bed. She has ruptured again! My brain computer takes only a split second to reach the conclusion this time, only five and a half hours after it initially strained so hard to reach the same conclusion.

This time we are not so lucky. As each stitch is replaced through the heart, it pulls through. Five-thirty and she is bleeding to death on the table with all of us standing silently, unable to pull it off again.

"Closing the hole the first time was difficult; closing it the second time was unbelievable; closing it the third time is impossible. She's dead." Dr. Bell backs away from the table and walks out of the room.

I remain, with blood still dripping from the operating table onto the floor, the front of my scrub suit soaked and with so much blood in my canvas operating shoes, I feel that now familiar squish when I move my feet. I begin closing the chest with one layer of heavy suture material—no use doing a plastic closure now. This is one wound which will never heal. I begin having far-reaching thoughts as I stand alone at the table closing the chest of a dead patient. "So this is the way I learn." This is the "I have to go through myself" experience necessary to acquire the knowledge of a chest surgeon. Learn by doing. Learn by seeing. "I would rather not have to learn this," I think to myself. We started the initial operation almost twenty-four hours ago and gave our all, yet she is dead and there is nothing we can do about it. No one is paying much attention to the fact that there is still a patient in the room. The scrub nurses are busy cleaning their tables and discussing what cases they are going to scrub on this morning. The anesthesiologist is cleaning his cart and replacing the drugs he has used. I hear an occasional laugh and a few complaints about the loss of sleep tonight just because of the chest doctors. I continue to sew, speaking only to my mind.

"She didn't have much of a chance either way," I think. "All chances are gone now. If we hadn't operated, she would be alive this very minute . . . but if she were alive, she couldn't do anything but get out of bed a few minutes a day." My brain argues with itself as I finish closing the chest. I place the last stitch. Time to forget Mrs. Krozier. A new day is here. This morning I am scheduled to put my first mitral prosthesis in a good-risk patient. I must put all my thoughts into that operation. I have to see if everything is in order for the procedure, need to make rounds on the patients still in I.C.U., and need to give instructions to the two patients to be discharged this morning.

Only as I remove my breakfast of cheese crackers from the snack machine and start toward the Coke machine do I realize I have not eaten for almost twenty-four hours. Even now, I am not hungry, only shaky from low blood sugar. Excitement replaces hunger but has no nourishment. There's no time to go through the cafeteria line.

One hour passes and I am busy with the normal workings of being chief resident. The incident which happened only hours ago seems weeks away—forgotten, too many things going on to think about that now. Forget the dead and concentrate on the living. I am experiencing—and learning. Perhaps this is the only way to get through my year as chief resident—concentrate on the living.

The mitral valve operation goes well today. I put in my first artificial valve but have no feeling of elation. I am numb to my surroundings. Mrs. Krozier died. Forgotten? Not quite. I performed a successful operation. It almost seems to emotionally balance out. A plus and a minus within a twenty-four hour period, and I find it difficult to cope with these feelings. I decide to go home for a while during the evening lull, but don't feel like telling Harriet I put my first valve in today. What's the use? Why keep going at this pace? What good is helping one person if the next one dies? I need some sleep to clear my mind enough to get back in there swinging. I decide not to eat supper, only to lie down on the sofa and snooze until the junior resident calls the latest lab results to me. Tomorrow will be better. I flip through my worn goal's book. I would hate to relive each experience that has led to an entry in the book. In some ways, it has been a terrible existence. In another way, it has been simply great; operating, operating, operating. It has been tremendous to be given the opportunity to train to become a surgeon, to experience all these situations which have made the *Goal's Rule Book* possible.

I close the notebook and relax.

The next day is brighter. Bob First, who worked under me as a resident on general surgery, starts his rotation on C-T as the junior resident. He has decided to go into cardio-thoracic and will stay on the service for the remainder of the year as my junior resident. He has already proven to be a hard, conscientious worker I can rely on, and his presence on the service makes a whole new world to work in. I am glad he decided on C-T, for he will be an asset to the inner workings of the program.

Bob and I decide we need a room near the I.C.U. that we can call home for awhile. We find a storage closet that is easily converted and dress it up a little. We talk the secretary into typing a copy of Murphy's Laws to tape to the wall of our new hangout. They seem so appropriate to our troubles:

1. In Any Field Of Scientific Endeavor, Anything That Can Go Wrong Will Go Wrong.
2. Left To Themselves, Things Always Go From Bad To Worse.
3. If There Is A Possibility Of Several Things Going Wrong, The One That Will Go Wrong Is The One That Will Do The Most Damage.
4. Nature Always Sides With The Hidden Flaw.
5. If Everything Seems To Be Going Well, You Have Obviously Overlooked Something.

The original plan for the interns and residents seems to be working. The intern on call will still remain in the I.C.U. throughout the night while Bob and I will be next door in our new on-call room. If a problem arises, the intern can come get the appropriate resident. Bob will handle most problems and will usually be called first. If he is unsure what to do, he will call me. There is only one problem—no beds. We borrow one from the pediatric on-call room since they have an extra, and we also find an old two-cushion sofa which can pass for a place to curl up. We are set.

It is strange that such a small thing as a room next to I.C.U. could make such a difference, but the entire service becomes more relaxed. Even the interns are satisfied, because now they don't have to fight Bob any more for the red easy chair in I.C.U.—a favorite place for all for a quick nap.

The past few days have been relatively easy with only scheduled surgery being performed. The emergency operations have been slack. When we are tied up with many emergencies our schedule can become completely turned upside down. If an emergency comes in at two in the morning, that is the time he has to be worked up and operated on. Without doubt, there are numerous times an emergency operation is required to save a life. Death has no timetable unless perhaps it is favorable to the nights when residents are trying to sleep.

I am awakened to the dreaded ringing of the phone and told there was a baby born yesterday afternoon with aortic stenosis, and she has just been transferred to the pediatric service nearly dead. We take her to the operating room immediately in an attempt to open the valve to relieve the pressure being built up within the heart. I am to be first surgeon. I don't understand. The baby is almost dead. One of the main valves in the heart is plugged. An emergency operation is about to be done, and I have been appointed first surgeon by Dr. Bell. I have advanced a rung on the ladder of becoming a surgeon. Emergencies do not allow for mistakes, and I am about to perform *my first cardiac emergency*. One stitch at a time is adding up. One brick at a time is at the top floor of the skyscraper, one stitch at a time is nearing the completion of the operation.

I discuss the procedure with Dr. Bell.

"The only chance the baby has is to take a Brock's valvulotome and push it through the valve opening and hope it works." Dr. Bell hastily makes ready for the operation by going over the valvulotome with me. "It's just like a small pencil with little side blades attached to where the lead point would be located. The trick to the operation lies in the fact the blades protract and retract. You can set the dial and let them protract as far out as you like. With this baby, we will barely be able to open them but it's our only chance."

I suddenly realized why he is letting me be first surgeon on the case. It is not so much that I have become such a great surgeon so early in my cardiac training, but rather because it is a simple technical procedure that requires no special surgical skill other than sticking a "pencil" in the heart and blindly pushing it through the

— 172 —

aortic valve, plus the fact the baby will, in all likelihood, not live, no matter who pushes it through the valve.

I expose the heart, such a miniature heart, and place a purse-string suture near the tip of the heart. Next, I stab the center of the hole I have just outlined with the suture. Now, the valvulotome. I gently push it through the opening I have just made. I grasp it with my right hand and push my left index finger on the base of the aorta and invaginate it momentarily—all I have to do is aim for my finger tip.

Set the dial to protract the blades.

Push. Through the valve.

Close the blades.

Pull. Back into the ventricle.

Remove the valvulotome from the heart.

Blood squirts through the hole in the heart.

Quickly tie the purse strings. Bleeding stops.

Close the chest . . . the baby is still alive.

There is immediate improvement, but she probably has had too much of a strain on the heart muscle to survive through the night.

She does survive, however, and two weeks later is discharged from the hospital. I feel good but not elated. I do not fully understand why I don't feel like a hero. Why am I not more proud? Probably because I acknowledge the fact I had very little control over what happened. I didn't even have faith the baby would make it through the first night much less be able to leave the hospital in two weeks.

Bob is enjoying the service since I am splitting the lung cases with him. We both want to learn as much as possible about surgery on the lung since a great deal of our surgical practice in the future will be centered on lung operations. This aspect of the cardio-thoracic surgery training is not as rewarding as the heart surgery, since so many of the patients with cancer of the lung are in a terminal state when we first see them. Patients are usually men who smoke one or two packs of cigarettes a day and then come to see us, worried about getting cancer.

They cannot grasp the reality that smoking causes cancer of the lung, and the more they smoke, the more of a chance they have of getting a tumor. I even try to get a patient who smokes three packs a day to make a wager with me on his chances of eventually dying of cancer of the lung. No one will take me up on the bet, but no one will quit smoking the three packs a day either. Lung cancer in women is on the rise, and the most obvious reason is that more women are smoking today than they did twenty-five years ago. Try to explain that to a nice-looking college co-ed student who has made up her mind that smoking is "the thing" to do, and see if it makes the slightest impression on her. The answer is "no."

We will always have patients who continue to smoke to excess until they "grow" their lung cancer and then decide to quit smoking a week before surgery in hopes it will make a difference on the outcome of life versus death.

Mr. Frank Harris is being admitted to the hospital today to our service for a routine work-up of lung cancer. After spending thirty minutes with him and reviewing his x-rays, I get the history that he has had a bad cough for several years and thought nothing about it until one morning when he noticed there were some small flakes of blood mixed with the mucus. He dismissed it completely, but a few weeks later the same thing recurred. He mentioned it to his wife, who immediately made an appointment for him to be examined. His local physician saw him, had a x-ray taken, and referred him to our service. There is a mass the size of a lemon in his right lung.

The first inquiry I make of the patient is whether there are some old x-rays for comparison that he may have had taken within the past few years. If he had a film taken five years ago and the spot was present then, and unchanged since then, there would be no need to operate just to take out something that isn't causing him difficulty and has almost no chance of being cancer. Mr. Harris has not had any chest films taken, however, so we are going to work him up from scratch. The work-up is begun by giving him a cup to spit into in the morning; the material will be examined under the microscope in search for malignant cells that can be "shedding" from the mass in his lung and be washed out in his sputum.

No malignant cells are found in his sputum.

Next is bronchoscopy, the process of passing a flexible lighted tube through the nose down the inside of the trachea and into his lung to look for the tumor. The bronchoscope is introduced into the larynx and windpipe, slid first down the larger air passage of each lung and eventually into the area where the mass is located. If any portion of the mass can be seen from "inside" the lung, a small piece is biopsied and sent to the pathologist for diagnosis. If nothing is seen, saline is injected into the bronchoscope and then suctioned back out. The material obtained in this manner is also sent to pathology in the hope that some of the cells have been washed off the tumor, allowing a diagnosis to be made.

Bob slides the bronchoscope neatly into the area of lung in which the tumor is located. The bronchi appear clearly. He slides in a small wire with a miniature brush on the end and pushes it on out the passage way beyond where he can see in hopes the brush will either penetrate the actual tumor or brush up against it and scrape some of the tumor cells onto the brush. The brush is sent to the pathologist to be looked at under the microscope.

Still no tumor cells; no diagnosis.

Due to the location of the mass on x-ray, there is a possibility that some of the tumor has spread into the lymph nodes up along the trachea. We decide to perform a mediastinoscopy, which entails making a small incision in Mr. Harris's neck and sliding a small, lighted, metal tube down alongside the trachea and bronchi. In this manner, the lymph nodes can be visualized and biopsies made to see if the tumor has spread to this area. If it has, the chances of curing him by surgery are very slim.

I perform the mediastinoscopy, visualize several lymph nodes, make biopsies and Mr. Harris returns to his room to await the pathologist's report.

The report comes back completely negative; no tumor seen on bronchoscopy, no tumor cells in the bronchoscopy washings, no tumor cells found in his sputum, and no tumor in any of the lymph nodes biopsied on mediastinoscopy. The only way left to determine if the spot on x-ray is cancer is to open his chest and actually take a piece of the mass and let the pathologist decide at that time.

Mr. Harris is scheduled for morning surgery. I position him on the operating table so that his right side is up. He is prepped and draped, and I make an incision through the skin beginning just under his right nipple and extend it backward, curving under his shoulder blade. The chest incisions are extensive by necessity to get the chest opened enough to have good visualization during the operation. The muscles of the chest wall are divided and the chest cavity itself is entered between the fourth and fifth ribs. Even though the muscles between the ribs are incised, the ribs remain in the same position as always; they have to be pried apart with a heavy metal gadget that is slid between the two ribs to push them apart. The ribs are separated seven or eight inches in this manner, allowing me to see, as well as get my hands and instruments inside the cavity to work.

"He really has the 'black lung'," Bob says commenting on how black the lung appears as he assists me on the case. A normal lung is pink and clean looking, but a lung of a chronic smoker begins to turn darker and darker until it becomes black with the carbon the lungs have absorbed.

I place both hands into the wound and feel the tumor mass. The right lung is separated into three lobes, or divisions, and I can feel the mass sitting in the middle lobe, close to the connection of the other two lobes.

"The bad disease," I tell Bob as I continue to explore the area with my hands. I feel for spread of the tumor in the other lobes and also in the lymph nodes around the main airway. I feel several nodes near the main branches, but none with the firm, "stuck down" feel of cancer that has spread. "I think the only way to get it out is to do a radical 'pneumo' on him. I'll biopsy a piece of the tumor for the frozen section."

I pull my hand out of the chest and let Bob take a feel to see if he finds anything different, or has any suggestions to make. I tell him my decision to do a radical pneumonectomy—to remove the entire lung as well as the lymph nodes situated around the trachea and the right main air passages. If the tumor were situated further out in the middle lobe, it may have been possible to remove only one lobe and leave the remaining two. However, Mr. Harris's tumor is sitting right on the main air passages and no margin of safety is present. If we leave any tumor behind, it will prove fatal.

Bob agrees with my decision. I send a small slice of lung containing the tumor to the pathologist. He sends back the report: carcinoma, squamous cell. There is cancer present.

We start the radical dissection by incising the thin pleural covering lining the cavity of the chest. As I bring the dissection down toward the lung, I include the lymph nodes which would be in the path where the tumor would spread. Next we dissect around the vessels to the lung, and isolate the artery and veins. Finally, the dissection is completed and the cancerous lung is removed. A tube is placed through the chest wall and the wound is closed.

The resection completed, Mr. Harris is taken to the recovery room.

"What will you tell him about what you found?" Bob asks as we leave the recovery room. This is one of the first cancers of the lung Bob has scrubbed on and he wants to know what to tell a patient who has cancer.

"I would tell him exactly what I would want to know if I went to a surgeon with a spot on my lung and paid him to find out what it was. I think the only thing you can do is tell it to him straight and tell him what his chances are. If he doesn't want to accept that as fact, then it's up to him to deny it to himself and to anybody else he wishes."

"What if the family asks you not to tell him he has cancer or tells you to wait a few months to let him know what you found? It seems like half the families made such requests when I rotated through the cancer service on general surgery."

"I know exactly what you are talking about. In some of the cancer cases, the tumor has to be left behind and you know there is no way possible for the patient to survive the malignancy. I have had some families ask me not to tell the patient, or worse still, even actually lie to the patient about what I have found. I assume these families try to act as if nothing is wrong and attempt to lead a normal life, once the patient is sent home to await death. I know this cannot last long before the patient begins to grow suspicious of the whole setup and especially of the surgeon who explained the finding to him," I explain to Bob as he writes the post-op orders on Mr. Harris's chart.

I continue: "I first explain to the family that I am going to tell the patient that he does have cancer and whether I was able to remove it all. Very few families argue with that approach. Then I go ahead and tell the patient what I found during surgery. Now, with some patients I can be straightforward and with others not so straight. You have to make the decision with each patient differently."

With the orders written and the conversation ended, it is time to do another bronchoscopy and mediastinoscopy on a man admitted yesterday with a spot on his lung. I observe over Bob's shoulder as he glides the scope into the patient's trachea.

I enjoy working with Bob. He is inquisitive, and this requires me to arrange my thinking well enough to be able to explain and discuss with him. I take out the *Goal's Rule Book* from my pocket. I flip through the pages and realize I have already made habits from most of what I have written down. These habits have been formed by repetition. I automatically throw out negative thoughts as they enter my mind and replace them with positive ones. The bad apple rule has become habit. I still make my daily lists of things to do in order of importance; it is now habit to do it that way. I look at things that need to be done, see them as immediate action goals and relate them to the overall goal structure of my intermediate and major goals. It has become habit. Large problems are automatically broken down to small one stitch at a time items. And as a matter of fact, I am already seeing myself having finished cardiothoracic training. What was once difficult to achieve is becoming easier through habit. I return to my rule book less and less; I am developing good habits through repetition of the rules. My mind has taken the rules and planted them, nourished them and now is harvesting them in the form of habits. Suddenly a scripture I have heard numerous times becomes real: "As a man thinketh in his heart, so is he." I am becoming what I have kept on my mind for the past several years. Thought has become habit, has become character. My character as a surgeon has matured from thoughts on becoming a surgeon. The giant steps between my thoughts, and the character I have developed as a surgeon were achieved only by putting my thoughts into action—the all important immediate action goals.

As the weeks roll by, I find I am letting Bob do more and more of the lung cases and find myself actually enjoying assisting him in the surgery. In return, Dr. Bell is allowing me to perform more and more of the open-heart cases. I have been blessed with success on most of them but am quick to remind myself that Dr. Bell does the difficult ones and leaves the easy ones to me, the ones who are supposed to do well. Dr. Bell informs me of a new patient just admitted for surgery this week.

Mrs. Willis is fifty-nine years old, an obese woman who is so sincerely friendly, I wish I could have known her when I was a child, so that I might have learned some of her friendly ways. She has seven boys whose ages range from thirteen (her baby as she calls him) to twenty-seven. They all come to the hospital to be with their mother while she undergoes open-heart surgery. They need each other at a time like this. The father was killed in an automobile accident eight years ago. They are a very close family, jabbing at each other, kidding the "baby," laughing with their mother. They talk as a unit, act as a whole. None of the boys is married, it's just them and

Mom. Dr. Bell and I talk to her and the boys about the forthcoming operation. All of them accept it as a necessity and plan to take it in stride.

Mrs. Willis had rheumatic fever twenty years ago which left her mitral valve, the heart valve between the left atrium and the left ventricle, in a similar way a cancerous growth affects the body. The reaction to the infection has chewed at the edges of the valve. Dense scar tissue has invaded the body of the valve, making it like stiff cardboard which does not move with each beat of the heart as a soft pliable, normal valve does. This results in a leak in the left side of her pump. Not only will the valve not close properly, it is so scarred down that it obstructs the forward flow of blood which normally should pass through the valve with little effort. She has been in heart failure over a year but "could not leave the boys long enough to have it looked after." Now, she has a large, distended heart which is in chronic failure and will prove to be very difficult to get "off the pump"—the heart-lung machine.

"She'll be a difficult case, but I think she ought to do O.K.," Dr. Bell says after walking out of her room. "Do you want to do her? She ought to be easy to get the valve in place since she has such a large atrium."

I nod in the affirmative, hoping nothing goes wrong with this case. I am midway through the year as chief resident and have fourteen valves under my belt. I have had no deaths from a valve case, mainly because of the "good-risk" classification of my patients. Mrs. Willis definitely is not a good risk, but I feel confident in tackling this more difficult heart.

I speak spontaneously to Dr. Bell. "I don't think I could bear facing those boys if something went wrong. The young one asked me if it would be all right if he planned to play football with his team Friday night. I am sure they don't understand the seriousness of the operation."

"She will do all right," Dr. Bell responds assuringly. I just wish she didn't have so much calcium in her valve. We will review her heart studies on film and evaluate the valve once more.

The morning of the operation begins at six-thirty. Bob and the students are already making rounds. I go by and check the most recent post-op patients before putting on my scrub suit to get ready for the case. Mrs. Willis is supposed to be in the operating room at seven, but she isn't even in the entrance hall at five to seven.

"Who's bringing Mrs. Willis down?" I ask a nurse at the O.R. desk.

"We're short handed this morning, and I do not think anyone has gone after her yet."

"If you don't have someone to get the heart patients here by seven, let me know. I'll get them down myself. We can't hold up the whole team just because someone didn't show for work." I angrily pick up the phone and call the seventh floor.

"I'm sorry, but we just don't have enough help around here," the operating room nurse repeats, shuffling papers on her desk.

I finally get Bob on the phone: "Bring Mrs. Willis down. I'll meet you at the elevator."

I hang up and begin a brisk walk toward the elevators. "What a way to start off," I think to myself. "I'm going to perform open heart surgery and have to roll the patient to the operating room myself."

Bob and I succeed in getting the patient into the room and begin helping the anesthesiologist put in the I.V. lines. Three lines are placed; a long catheter in a vein in the left arm is threaded into one of the large veins emptying into the heart; two catheters threaded through needles are stuck into each jugular vein in the neck. One of these is passed into the superior vena cava, just above the heart and connected to a monitor to measure the pressure of the blood just before it enters the heart. Mrs. Willis is awake during all this but offers no hint of discomfort. Bob and I next perform a cut-down over the radial artery in her left wrist. The artery is partially divided and another catheter is inserted into the vessel for about one-half inch. This catheter is connected to yet another monitor which will record the blood pressure continuously while we are operating. Just to the right of the patient is the large black multi-monitor with numerous connections and lines running to the patient, including the two pressure lines we just placed. The technicians run the monitor, all important at critical times during the procedure. The top portion of the monitor consists of a screen in which the E.K.G., the venous pressure, and the arterial pressure repeatedly sweep across the face of the screen for easy interpretation by the surgeon and anesthesiologist while the patient is on the heart-lung machine.

On the left of the patient is the life sustaining heart-lung machine, which receives blood from the patient and pumps blood, rich in oxygen, back into the patient. Mrs. Willis is put to sleep. I open the chest and incise the pericardium, the thin sac around the heart. I spread the edges of the sac apart, revealing the glistening heart muscle. There are four chambers in the heart—the right atrium, the right ventricle, the left atrium, and the left ventricle. It is easier thinking of the heart as a two-sided organ; the right side receiving blood from the body and pumping it through the lungs and into the left side; the left side receiving the blood from the lungs and pumping it into the aorta and throughout the body. The heart-lung machine works on the idea of placing a siphon hose into the heart just where the blood is entering the first chamber, and stealing the blood from the "right heart" and giving it to the heart-lung machine. The machine, in turn, will supply this blood with oxygen, doing the work of the lungs, and then pump the oxygenated blood through another tube, doing the work of the left heart. The heart is completely bypassed and can be opened, cut on, sewn or patched all the while the body continues to thrive on the flow of blood coming from the miraculous heart-lung machine.

I place all the connecting tubes into Mrs. Willis' heart and pass them off the table to the technician running the heart-lung machine. He connects the tubes to his pump and after the entire system is filled with blood, turns on the pump which begins to push oxygen rich blood back into the body. The heart is completely bypassed and nearly empty of blood. I open the left atrium and examine the valve. The mitral valve appears exactly as we were afraid it would—so scarred with calcium it looks and feels like bone. The leaflets of the valve are firm, scarred, useless, and will certainly be difficult to remove. An attempt is made to excise the valve by cutting with scissors but this proves futile. A clamp, similar to needlenose pliers, is used to crush and chew at the calcified valve until it is broken enough to excise with a pair of heavy duty curved scissors.

Much time elapses in removing the valve. I begin sewing an artificial valve into position with difficulty. Nothing seems to be going right. The calcium does not stop at the base of the valve, but extends into the heart tissue where the stitches have to be placed to hold the artificial valve. The needles bend as I push them through this unsewable area, the sutures pull out when tied with any tension at all; it seems impossible to get the artificial valve into place.

Finally, after much frustration and difficulty, the valve is in and ready to be tested. We have spent several hours getting the valve removed and the prosthesis sewn in. The heart muscle itself is sick as a result of battling the diseased valve, and it will be short of a miracle if it survives this added insult of surgery. The heart-lung machine is turned off gradually and the heart is given an opportunity to take over the work it has been accustomed to for such a long time. It begins pumping some blood, but not enough and with inadequate force to profuse the organs of her body. We try everything in the book to aid this dying heart to beat effectively once again. Word is sent to her sons that their mother is not doing well in coming off bypass. We decide to once again open the heart to see if, by chance, the valve has pulled loose or is allowing blood to leak around the edges which may keep her from taking over again.

The valve looks just as we left it, firmly sewn in place. Her heart simply isn't strong enough to recover from the long operation and both Dr. Bell and I know it. One more attempt is made to get Mrs. Willis off bypass, but the heart muscle has been under too much stress for too many years to be put through the strain we just placed on it. Two more hours are spent trying to get her heart to take over.

"Turn off the pump, she's gone." Dr. Bell gives the order. I look at him, knowing the most difficult task is yet to be performed. I have been first surgeon, I am the one to tell the seven boys their mother is dead. I dread talking with them. No one in the room knows how I dread it, but it must be done.

"I'll go tell them." Not much else is said as I leave the room for the long walk down the corridor to the waiting room where the boys wait to hear any news about their mother. Several nurses speak to me as I meet them in the hallway, but I hardly notice them as I rehearse what to say. The nursing supervisor has placed them in a separate room adjacent to the waiting room. I walk in, shut the door behind me. Seven pairs of eyes stare into mine, and all remain motionless as if time has stopped, to wait for me to speak.

What do I say? Do I look at the floor? Do I look at the wall? Do I dare look at the boys? What can I say to make it seem less real? An hour of thoughts race through my mind in the brief moment before speaking.

"Boys, I am afraid she didn't make it. We tried everything, but couldn't get the heart to work." I look at the oldest. He fights to keep back the tears but soon his cheeks become moistened as he stands, eyes fixed upon mine, gently nodding his head.

"We knew it. We knew the minute we were told she wasn't doing well earlier. We knew it the way the nurse asked us to step in here. We knew it when you walked in and shut the door. Even though we knew it, we still had *hope* . . . until just now." His voice breaks as he turns and puts his arm around his youngest brother.

The young one whines at first, but soon begins sobbing. The other brothers grab each other for solace, and the oldest is able to thank me for trying before he sits down and buries his face in his hands.

All of the explanation in the world cannot change the fact that Mrs. Willis is dead, will never utter a sound, breathe a breath of air, or give a friendly greeting to her boys again. This is all that registers in the family's mind, all that matters to them. Yet, I must try to explain to myself what happened during the surgery, what went wrong, why she died. This, a surgeon has to do in order to ever be able to operate again. He cannot leave anything unanswered in his own mind; this is the one time he has to be honest with himself or loose his "right" to operate. Only *he* can know whether the best was done for the patient, whether death was preventable. It is a complicated problem that is never completely solved in anyone's mind. The family of the dead patient must live through this problem only once, but the surgeon must face this ever-present drama each and every time a patient dies.

I leave the room. I don't know why, but a single thought concerning the youngest comes into my mind. Today is Thursday. Tomorrow, all the high school players have their football game. All except one.

Death is a terrible situation for the family to face, but it is the most horrifying experience a resident will ever go through. Death is so final! There is no second chance at treatment. It is unbearably difficult to try to explain death on the operating table to the family when I can't even begin to understand it myself.

Death acquires the largest portion of hatred I can muster under any circumstances. I know I must pull away from the emotional aspect of a patient dying, but I really wonder if I will ever be able to. The prevention of death, almost at any cost, becomes instilled in our minds as each day of the residency progresses. I am sure there is a double exposure to this picture of death. One, the empathy felt with the family and two, even when the surgeon knows he has given the patient the best operation possible, there is always a feeling of insecurity, of doubt, of defeat, when the patient does not survive. I can only hope I don't have a series of Mrs. Willises to face.

*　　*　　*

I push on. Days turn to weeks, weeks to months. I become more proficient in running the service, and my confidence builds with each case we operate on. The hours are long but very rewarding. I become aware of a compulsive drive to work. I know this has developed over the years of surgical training, but only now I am aware of the way I do things. I have made myself strive for perfection, knowing the impossibility of the feat. I cannot explain it to myself, but I know I have realized some benefits from this attitude—intangible benefits, perhaps—but the overall gains in life cannot always be measured directly by whether we try harder on any particular feat or job, but they are measured indirectly by an overall mental attitude.

I will have to change before long. I cannot live life knowingly making myself compulsive, but must continue this frame of mind until the completion of residency. The program is far too pressing to tackle without an aggressive spirit. The *Goal's Rule Book* has been a valuable asset in getting as far as I have. The rules are easier and easier to apply to new situations. Life as a surgeon is becoming easier and more natural. I feel at home now.

However, there is a price paid for all this training. An amount that I do not know as of yet. This is the price of marriage. I am home very seldom, and Harriet is getting along in her pregnancy. I am not the supportive husband I should be during a time like this. We are not together enough to really call it "living together." We are pulling together, but do not seem to be making great headway. I am in a successful situation but what a price to have to pay. Harriet and I do not discuss it because we have both convinced ourselves that this pattern is only temporary. I hold on to that belief. How can a man help direct his children if he is never around to give direction? How can a man's wife continue to support him and care for him if he is never around to be loved? How can a marriage grow and mature in a situation like this? I have many questions, but few answers. I continue on "one stitch at a time."

The week finally ends, and on this particular Saturday morning I decide not to go to the M & M conference and spend the three-hour block in the anatomy room dissecting coronary arteries. I never miss this particular conference, but Dr. Bell is away and we won't be

discussing our complications or deaths. Time will be more benefi-
cially spent in the lab studying arteries of the heart. Thousands of
patients die each year from the blockage of these arteries that results
in myocardial infarctions (heart attacks). Surgery is being performed
by taking a segment of vein from the patient's leg and using it to
bypass the blocked area in the artery. One end of the vein is sewn
into the aorta, the other end is sutured into the artery in the heart
carrying blood around the blocked area. I decide the best way to
learn the anatomical details of these arteries is to follow them out
through an actual preserved heart.

I am just finishing dissection on the right coronary artery, when
the intern comes running into the anatomy room.

"Better hurry! A man just came into the E. R. who put a
shotgun to his chest and blew out the whole left side." I lay the heart
on the dissecting table and quickly follow him out of the room, not
taking time to wash the harsh, odorous formalin from my hands. We
run down the hall toward the operating room. There is so much
excitement in the intern's voice, he is almost shouting at me, too
excited to give many answers. I nod and keep running.

I enter the operating room without stopping to change into a
scrub suit. A man is lying on the operating table with blood pouring
out the left side of his chest, onto the table, and pooling on the floor.
The anesthesiologist is in the process of putting a tube in his
windpipe, and two scrub nurses are hastily opening gowns and
instruments.

I quickly glance around and realize I am the ranking surgeon in
the room, with the responsibility to save this patient. What should I
do? I am still in street clothes, standing in the midst of nurses,
interns, and residents who are scurrying around trying to get sterile
gowns and gloves on. All the while more and more blood pours out
of the patient's chest and pools on the floor. I have never been in
such a situation before. Thus far, nothing in training has taught me
what to do with a patient like this. No one in the room has taken any
definitive steps to alleviate the situation. There is no one here to
look to for advice. All I have is my "computer."

"Give me a knife!" One of the scrub nurses hands me a knife,
and I make an incision at opposite edges of the gaping hole in the
chest to give me room enough to get my hand in. Groping through
the blood filled cavity I feel for the hilum of the lung, the area
adjacent to the heart where the arteries come out of the heart and

enter the lung. The heart is hardly beating as I slide my hand down on the hilum in an attempt to get control of the bleeding. Spreading my two fingers apart, I am able to wedge the larger arteries in between them. I squeeze my fingers together, like closing a pair of scissors; the bleeding stops as if by some magical power. I now have time to evacuate the blood and clot to see what I have. The entire left lung is in bits and pieces.

"Give me the biggest clamp you have."

The nurse hands me a large DeBakey aneurysm clamp. I place it across the area I am holding between my fingers. The bleeding stops completely. The intern and anesthesiologist busily pump un-cross-matched blood into the patient who, by some act of fate, is still alive. In less than sixty seconds, the situation is under control. Blood is going into his system, none is coming out.

I have a feeling of accomplishment that is indescribable. I have been placed in a live or die situation and right now believe the results are going to be successful. Even though I have never even thought about what to do in such a situation, I assessed it correctly and acted accordingly. This has to be one of the peaks in my training.

However, I am only one-tenth finished with the operation that faces me. He has not been prepped and has not been draped. I am still in my street clothes, and blood is everywhere. I accept a gown and gloves and we clean and formally drape the patient. Assessing the situation in the chest, I observe that he has blown most of his left lung out but has caused very little damage to his heart. The remaining bits and pieces of his left lung will have to be removed and a cover has to be made for the big hole the shotgun left in his chest wall. The remainder of the operation proves to be straightforward; by the time we finish, his blood pressure is stable and it becomes evident we have saved his life.

After the case, I shower and change into a clean scrub suit that I will wear home since my clothes are so bloody. I sit alone in the dressing room and think about a subject I have thought about before. Why do so much to save someone who has just tried to kill himself? His last wish was to die and not have to face reality. Now, I have denied him a wish so strong that he would put a shotgun to his chest and pull the trigger. The problem that made him pull the trigger will still be there in the morning, plus he will realize he was even a failure in ending his own life. Will he ever be grateful that he was unsuccessful? These are questions I cannot answer. I suppose he will answer them for me by either trying it again or thanking me for my efforts.

I also reflect back to my initial actions in the operating room. There were other residents and doctors in the emergency room when the patient came in. There were more physicians in the operating room. Yet, no definitive action had been taken to stop the bleeding. Could the rule of immediate action goals have applied here? Is it possible that I have trained my mind to go ahead and act now on the immediate goal of getting the bleeding stopped? Perhaps the *Goal's Rule Book* is paying off in important dividends that I do not even realize.

Three weeks later, I discharge the patient from the hospital. He says he is grateful for what I have done, but I don't really know how sincere his gratitude is. Neither do I know if the next suicide attempt will feel any appreciation for my services, but I know I will do everything in my power to give him that choice.

I get a few minutes to go over some thoughts on cardiac surgery with a handful of students who are sitting in our on-call room next to the I.C.U. One of them asks about the future of heart surgery. I reply: "As time passes, I become more and more intrigued with the possibilities that await the future of surgery on the heart. It is interesting to read the history of this field and realize how much progress has been made relatively recently. Surgeons and cardiologists alike have been interested for years in getting more blood flow to a heart that is ischemic—one not getting enough blood flow through blocked arteries. As far back as the mid-thirties, attempts were made to bring the "fatty apron," the omentum, out of the abdomen and sew it against the outside of the heart muscle in hopes that some of the blood supply of the omentum would creep across and also supply the heart muscle. I learn that in the mid-forties an artery in the chest was "tunneled" into the diseased heart muscle and actually improved the symptoms in a significant number of patients. However, the most interesting aspect of this new field began in 1958 with the introduction of actually injecting dye into the arteries of the heart and taking motion pictures with x-ray film in order to visualize blocks in the arteries to see which of the three main arteries of the heart needed to be carrying more blood. This technique opened the door to a new field of surgery on the heart.

"If you obtain a heart from the anatomy department and complete the dissection of the coronary arteries, you can correlate what you actually see in the inner walls with what you read concerning the disease process that goes on inside these arteries. They are being choked with plaques that leave the inner linings looking much like a clogged up drainage pipe. The difference in appearance of the arteries and the pipe is mainly that the lining of the arteries are firm and covered with a smooth layer of tissue. However, the end result of both are the same—plugging the opening and preventing any flow through the pipe or artery.

"These patients with partially or completely blocked vessels usually exhibit the symptoms of angina pectoris—a squeezing, pressure-like chest pain that is commonly described as a tightness or pressing sensation felt behind the sternum. It is usually not well localized and can radiate to other portions of the body, mainly the left shoulder or down the left arm. This pain is brought on when the patient exerts himself and can usually be relieved by the patient stopping and resting.

"Some of these patients can benefit from a better supply of blood to the heart, past the area of blockage in the artery. After a patient has been studied by the dye injected in his arteries and does become a candidate for surgery, a vein can be removed from his leg and one end sewn into the aorta, and the other end of the vein sewn into the artery in the heart, at a site past the blockage."

The discussions with the students completed, I am reminded we have a coronary bypass patient being admitted today. He has already been extensively studied by the cardiologists and has been referred to us for coronary artery bypass.

"Why don't all of you go by the lab and see what his studies show?"

Joe Howard is the patient and I find he has "three vessel disease." Each of the three main arteries in his heart is blocked to some degree, meaning the operation will be more of a risk, more difficult to perform, and the chances of a "cure" less than if he had only one vessel partially blocked with the other two branches open. Dr. Bell tells me the prognosis is even worse in Joe's case because his heart function is so borderline; it stopped beating on the cardiac catheterization table when the dye was injected into the coronary arteries during the coronary arteriograms. His heart is so starved for blood that the few moments the dye was mixed with the blood going to the heart was enough to make his heart stop beating; a very unusual event.

I walk into Joe's room and introduce myself. Joe is slightly obese, forty-four years old, covered with black hair, literally, from head to toe. He has so much hair on his chest that it looks as if he has on a black wool sweater as he removes his shirt for me to examine him. His wife is with him.

"I saw Dr. Billings and I told him I am going to will my body for his students to cut on if I don't make it." He greets me with this statement straightforwardly and in all sincerity. Dr. Billings is head of the anatomy department in the medical school and is a close friend of Joe's, and evidently Joe has discussed the possibility of donating his body to the school. Both Joe and his wife seem to sense the possibility of death more than any other patient I have ever taken care of.

"Well, we certainly won't think along those lines, Joe. Besides, you have too nice a wife to even be thinking such thoughts." Joe's wife is a very pretty woman with olive skin who wears her silky black hair tied at the back of her head. She is a "young" thirty-eight and seems the epitome of sophistication sitting in the red vinyl stuffed chair beside Joe's bed.

"My chances aren't so good, are they, Doc?"

I attempt to imagine what it is like to be in Joe's place as he speaks to me. His chances aren't so good and he is intelligent enough to realize this. There is to be no small talk with him. He knows the name of the game and knows the cards he is holding. He has been dealt a bum hand. If I were in his shoes, could I talk about the possibility of death as freely as Joe? Could I really admit the fact the odds were stacked high against me? Some people in a similar situation talk this way just to get the doctor to give them words of encouragement, but I sense that Joe is talking because this actually is on his mind—just as he is spilling it out to me.

"Joe, I am sure the operation and the risks of the surgery have been discussed with you in detail by Dr. Bell. He will be with us on evening rounds. He'll discuss that with you."

I am still uneasy discussing the risk of surgery with a patient as frank and straightforward as Joe, and I elect to take the easy way out and refer such discussions to Dr. Bell. I acknowledge to myself that before my training is complete, I will need to be able to discuss all possible complications following surgery. I must learn more than just how to perform operations.

Day One: The day for the operation arrives, all of Joe's questions will soon be answered. I assist Dr. Bell in the operation. I make an incision in the right leg, start removing the vein we will use in the bypass portion of the procedure. While doing this, Dr. Bell splits the sternum and opens the pericardial sac surrounding the heart in preparation for the bypass. Dr. Bell takes the vein I have removed and cuts it into three segments and meticulously sews each segment into the aorta and into each of the coronary arteries. Soon there is good flow to the vessels of the heart, the operation is completed and tubes are placed through the chest wall and into the operative area in order to drain the oozing blood that will follow surgery. Joe is taken to the recovery room for three hours and then taken to the intensive care unit. He has just survived the most critical early postoperative hours. He goes through the night with no unusual occurrences. His wife still wearing a black dress remains all night waiting patiently outside the unit.

Day Two: We are all pleased Joe has come through so well. One thing bothers us though. All of his studies are borderline normal. He is slow coming around, doesn't want to eat, doesn't want to get out of bed, doesn't want to talk to anyone, will not laugh; all in all, he has become a number one grouch.

Day Three: Status quo.

Day Four: He begins developing some lung complications.

Day Five: It becomes evident by evening he has pneumonia and is having difficulty keeping his oxygen saturation within a normal limit. The intern and I discuss Joe's complications as I glance rather methodically at the cardiac monitor at the foot of Joe's bed. The monitor is running twenty-four hours a day, and it is my habit to examine the squiggling lines as they race across the screen. Very seldom do I actually witness a significant change in the rhythm of the heart on the monitor, but I realize it is presently changing before my eyes. *Right now* something is happening to Joe's heart. Ventricular fibrillation! The ventricles are only quivering ineffectively and give a cardiac tracing on the monitor as if a nervous individual were trying to draw a straight line. We immediately begin resuscitation, including external cardiac massage. A piece of plywood is placed under Joe's back for support, and I put the heel of my hands on his sternum and begin pushing. Each time I push the sternum down, it is pushed against the heart and the grafts. I am sure such trauma can clot them off or even tear them loose.

The heart is shocked electrically and a breathing tube is placed into his windpipe. We get him back to a regular rhythm, but I have no idea what damage has been done to the vein grafts as a result of all the pounding during closed chest massage. At least he is still alive and now back to a regular rhythm. A successful outcome will be long in coming.

I walk out to the waiting room to tell Joe's wife what has happened. She is sitting in the lounge with a light blanket pulled around her legs. She has been able to catch a few cat naps earlier in the night but is reading a book as I approach. I had talked her into going to a friend's house last night in order to get some sleep, but she insisted, for some reason, on staying at the hospital this particular evening. She also insists on wearing a black dress. I'm not sure what this does for Joe's morale, but I wish she would wear something red, or blue, or anything but these black dresses. She looks startled and apprehensive as I approach her. She did not hear the ever dreadful "Code 500, intensive care unit; Code 500," which the relatives of patients in I.C.U. find out means something drastic is happening and all available doctors in the hospital are to report to the unit. There was no such call in this instance since we were at his bed at the time of fibrillation and there was no need for further help. She is sure she would have heard such a page if anything had happened to Joe. This only makes it more difficult to explain that something has happened to her husband.

"I am sorry to have to tell you, but Joe has had a setback. His heart quit beating momentarily, and we had to give him external massage and place him on a respirator. He is holding his own now, but I am not sure where this is going to lead us. We will continue to do everything possible for him and hope for the best." She does not rise as I tell her of the situation. She only nods and stares at the floor.

"I will be all right. I would like to be left alone right now." She continues to stare at the floor. I feel awkward as I stand over her. I want to say more, to tell her he is alive and we have that to be thankful for; that she will be able to go in and see him in a few minutes and actually talk to him; that this doesn't mean that he is going to die—that he still has a chance to make it. But there is a "sense" in the air that she will not accept any of these statements, that she knows his odds of living now have just dropped from forty percent to ten percent, that there is no use kidding herself as to what has happened.

"You can come in and see him if you like." I turn and walk back toward the unit. Her mood is so "thick" I feel almost reverent as I leave her sitting by herself. I stay by Joe's bed for the remainder of the night. She never comes to see him while I am there.

Day Six: Joe continues to slide downhill.

Day Seven: I do a tracheostomy in order to suction the secretions from his lungs and try to get at his pneumonia.

Day Ten: Still alive but vascular status unstable.

Day Fifteen: Persistent pneumonia requiring therapeutic bronchoscopy four times per day.

Day Eighteen: Pneumonia worse. Blood gases inadequate for survival. On respirator.

Day Twenty-one: Worse.

Day Twenty-three: Joe dies.

I talk with his wife. We have come to know each other in a unique way during these twenty-three days. Yes, she will permit an autopsy to be performed—if for no other reason than to let us know what went wrong. Yes, she still wants his body to go to the anatomy department. Joe wanted it that way. No, she never thought he would live through the operation; in her mind he died twenty-three days ago. She will grieve her husband's death and will find it difficult to explain to her children. She thanks me for my consideration, for keeping her informed of what was going on. I finally understand why she always wore the black dresses—she was mourning her husband from the time he came into the hospital.

I never see her again but think of her from time to time over the next few days whenever I see an attractive young woman wearing a black dress. On such occasions, I have to keep my mind from wandering back into the thoughts of the losing battle of those twenty-three days with Joe.

Three weeks later, I have all but forgotten Joe Howard as I stroll through the anatomy lab. One of the students recognizes me and yells across the room, "Say, you ought to remember this one. You all did him in, didn't you?" He jokingly motions me toward his table. I glance his way and recognize the hairy body on the dissecting table. They are dissecting Joe's right leg. There is one vein missing, but I don't feel like explaining to them why it isn't there, that it was removed in a futile operation. I don't feel like explaining anything to them, not even why I am ignoring his comment and am walking on out the lab.

I am grateful things are slack. After going through the anatomy lab, I don't feel much like doing anything. The *Goal's Rule Book* is no help now. Just keep going, keep working, quit thinking.

I go by the office to pick up the consultation sheets from the medicine department. I pull out the familiar blue slips marked "C-T Surgery." There are more than the usual amount for one day.

Looking at the consultation sheets I see a pediatric heart patient, a lung abscess, a carcinoma of the lung, and one sheet on a Mr. McLaughlin, who has a bad aortic valve in his heart. It says he may need an emergency valve replacement.

They've done it again. Mr. McLaughlin needed his valve replaced a year ago, and they treated him medically so long that we are going to have to do it with him half dead. They didn't even call me about him, but sent a blue slip to be picked up when I got around to it; I'd better go see him.

Mr. McLaughlin is dying. There is no way to save him by operating on him. I'll present him to Dr. Bell. I know he will operate as a last ditch effort. Not one patient in twenty will survive under these conditions. If we spend just ten hours at the operating table on these extreme-risk patients, that would amount to two hundred hours of surgery alone, to possibly save one patient. Not only that, but ten times that amount of time is spent after the operation to try to keep them alive and they still die. Two years earlier, he would have been a straightforward case and have been out of the hospital in ten days.

Still, we owe this to each patient. We are not mechanics who can pick and choose the job wanted, but are morally obligated to give this patient his one chance in twenty of surviving. This is Dr. Bell's philosophy, which results in his spending a significant amount of time on these extremely poor risk patients. He will never increase his batting average operating on patients like Mr. McLaughlin.

We cut. Six hours later, we cannot get him off the pump. His heart will not take over. He is dead. I angrily blame the medicine department for not referring him to us sooner, but Dr. Bell informs me Mr. McLaughlin refused surgery for six months. It was his own decision.

There is little to do this afternoon since our patient died on the table. I look forward to not having the strain of keeping a close check on a post-op patient for a change. A resident from the O.B. department pages me. Like a light switch going on, I know what is happening: Harriet must be in labor. I answer the page.

"Your wife is here and having good contractions. Dr. Ellison wants to know if you still want her to have epidural spinal anesthesia.

"That's what she said she wanted. Go ahead and start it. I'll be right over." Boy, this is exciting! I can't believe that she is actually going to deliver in the daytime and at a time when I am not so busy that I cannot be with her some.

The epidural is already in when I arrive in her labor room. She looks relaxed and flashes a big smile for me.

I gently rub her abdomen. "What are we going to have?"

"We'll know as soon as a few more of these contractions come, and I don't think it will be long."

Dr. Ellison comes in. He is a big man, authoritative. "Do you want to watch your little wife put this baby out?"

"No sir. I'll just wait and let you tell me what it is and how it went."

I go out to the desk and wait while they take Harriet into the delivery room. I just hope nothing goes wrong. I pick up a pencil and make some dots on the paper on the desk. Then I try to place the point of the pencil exactly on each dot, just to prove to myself that my hands are not shaky, that I am staying calm. Some of the dots are difficult to hit.

"Girl. Both did well. Congratulations." Dr. Ellison is off to another patient.

Father of two! Harriet did well. Her name is Patricia. Harriet named her when she first became pregnant. I wonder how she knew we would have a girl?

The night brings good sleep. Patricia. It feels good going to sleep thinking about a little baby two floors up named Patricia.

I get a decent night's sleep and awaken early to begin the routine once more. We have another heart to do today. It doesn't take long to forget about patients we have lost a few hours ago and get back into the swing of operations all day long. It is more difficult to forget about Harriet and Patricia, but I force myself to think into the future—not a year from now, not a week, but only a few hours at a time. A slight smile creeps onto my face as I think back to one of the rules I made as an intern. One stitch at a time. It works. This residency is passing a day at a time but it will be over some day. The major goal will be reached. Not in one day but in successfully completing one immediate action goal after another. It is about to fall in place and it's the greatest feeling in the world.

Today's heart case goes well, and the post-op care isn't as time-consuming as most cases. However, a late, leaking aneurysm keeps us up the best part of the night.

I check on Harriet before retiring for the night. She gets to go home in the morning. Bob and I retire to our "suite" for a coffee break. I am not sure what causes moods to change, but, for some reason, after working all day and into the night, there is something almost mystical about opening the window and letting cool night air in while lounging back on the bed and beginning a discussion on thought-provoking subjects. I lie back on the bed while Bob stretches out on some cushions on the floor.

"What do you think of euthanasia?" Bob asks. "Do you think there is ever a time we ought to decide a person should die when there is no hope whatsoever; or even one step further, actually terminate his life some way?"

He is serious about his questioning. I begin to answer: "That is a thought that enters the mind of every doctor who has treated a patient with a terminal disease who is within a few days or hours of dying. It is just natural instinct to keep doing everything possible to keep a patient alive, just as it is a natural instinct not to want to be defeated by death. Where is the line drawn between good patient care and personal defeat? Where is the line drawn between whipping a dead horse and considering the fact the patient's family has now spent all its savings and is starting to borrow money to pay the bills. The family would sell everything they owned to do this, but is it fair to the patient who has spent his entire life earning and saving money so that his wife and children may have the necessities of life after he has left them? But the physician reminds himself, 'this is the only and last chance this patient will ever have to get well, and life is certainly worth more than all the money in the world.' So both sides of the coin continue to turn up." I stop for a minute to check Bob to see if he has fallen asleep. Neither of us usually looks at the other during such discussions, and it is not unusual for the listener to fall asleep. Bob is relaxed but not asleep.

"You really expect me to give you an answer, do you?" I reposition onto my back, putting my hands behind my head and gaze once more at the ceiling. I want to get comfortable before going into my long dissertation on the subject.

"O.K., Bob, I'll give you three patients. I'll tell you what I did on the first two and let you tell me what to do on the third.

"The first was a twenty-year-old woman I was called to see on the medicine service earlier this year. She had trouble with a pregnancy and ended up with a tracheostomy. She was out of it completely for about two weeks and then came around, became alert, could breathe on her own, and the tracheostomy tube was removed. I was called to see her two weeks later and found her barely able to ventilate air in and out of her lungs. She was in a terrible state of anxiety because she knew she was suffocating and would not be able to last much longer. There was no thought process for me to go through to decide whether to try to save this patient or not. This was a clear-cut case—do an emergency tracheostomy since the trachea had scarred from the previous tracheostomy. So much scar tissue had formed, it was blocking the passage of air through her trachea. I later resected the scarred area and reconnected the remaining trachea."

"Come on, get down to it." Bob is impatient after hearing such a straightforward case. There is no question in his mind that he would have done the same thing.

"O.K., the second one came in last year on general. An old lady about seventy years old had an arterial bypass placed from her aorta down to her thighs because her legs weren't getting enough blood. This operation was performed about six weeks before I saw her in the emergency room. Whoever operated on her had put a Dacron tube from her thigh to her knee. Blood flow was O.K. through the graft, but the wound in her thigh became infected. The graft suddenly pulled loose, and she started pouring blood from it. She came into the E.R. in shock, but was still conscious enough to know what was going on. I got a clamp on the artery and began to explain to her that we were going to take her to the operating room and 'fix her up.' I was explaining what we would have to do when she instructed me to let her die. I told her that was ridiculous, to get that reasoning out of her mind, that she was going to be all right. She looked right at me again and repeated that she was ready to die. There was no doubt in the sincerity of this request. I didn't know what to say. Her sister had brought her to the hospital and was waiting in the hall, so I went out to see if she could talk some sense into this 'youngster.' In the meantime I ordered six units of blood typed and cross-matched and told the operating room to get ready for an emergency operation.

"I confronted her sister with what I had been told. She just smiled and nodded. She went on to explain the hours the two had discussed what should be done if a complication did occur and they had come to the agreed upon conclusion. 'She's been through so much.' She told me, 'There's just the two of us, and one of us has to go before the other.' She kept talking like this, and I soon realized that they had been very orderly and thorough in reaching the decision to 'pass on quietly.'

"You should have seen everybody jump me when I canceled the order for the blood and sent her to a private room on the fifth floor and told the nurses not to go into the room. Her sister sat with her for the remaining three hours of her life.

"Bob, are you awake?" I look over and see Bob with his eyes closed and head against the cushion on the floor.

"Yes, I'm awake," he replies. "I was in on that case with you and agreed with your decision at the time. Don't you remember anything?"

"Why didn't you stop me before I went through the whole story."

"Thought I'd see if you would tell it right. Now give me the problem case before we have to check I.C.U. again."

"O.K. This is one I had before you came on the service, and I guarantee it's a hard one." I settle back on the bed once more and begin to tell of a tragic case of six months ago.

"A forty-seven-year-old woman with a non-resectable tumor in her windpipe for which she had been given cobalt treatments. She continued to gasp for every breath, so I took her to the O. R. and did a tracheostomy. The tumor was located below the tracheostomy site, so I took a flexible tube and pushed through the tracheostomy, cramming it past the tumor. You have the picture now. Woman with a tumor, can't breathe, can't talk, tracheostomy done, tube pushed through tracheostomy and past the tumor mass. She can breathe through the tube, feels good, wants to go home."

"I get the picture. What did you do?" Bob's eyes are now open but he stares at the ceiling.

"As you know, the tumor would continue to grow, and if it didn't pinch the tube closed, lung secretions would eventually block it off. Now, you can keep her in the hospital and keep the secretions suctioned out and she will enjoy a few days with her family and then the tube plugs off and she dies. Or, you could not have done the tracheostomy in the first place and watched her suffocate over five or six days. Or, you could have given her an injection to sedate her to the point she would quit fighting for air. Or, you could actually prevent her from breathing—true euthanasia."

Bob rolls over and looks at me. "That's simple. Don't do the tracheostomy in the first place. Let her get death over with. She's going to be scared of that tube you stuck in her for the rest of her life. She won't enjoy the life you save for her."

"I keep thinking of that but it seemed cruel at the time. Come on; it's time to get some more blood gases. Tell you what. Since you're so smart, why don't you get the gases and I'll take a nap."

Bob slowly gets off the floor and heads for the door. "I know you aren't going to tell me what you ended up doing, and I'm not going to ask you to tell me. Frankly, I don't know if I could hold back and not do a tracheostomy and let the patient live awhile and then die that way or not. If ever that happens to me, just go ahead and shoot me." Bob leaves the room and heads for the I.C.U.

I lie with my eyes closed and feel my mind slowly sinking into the bottomless pit of darkness and restful sleep. I start wondering why I did the tracheostomy in the first place. She would have literally drowned in her own secretions and suffocated if I had not done it. But it would have been slow. However, she would have to face a similar death a few weeks later, even with the tracheostomy in. "It just seemed the thing to do at the time. I just seemed . . ." Sleep comes easily when it comes so infrequently.

I end up with four hours of uninterrupted sleep while Bob obtains three frequently interrupted hours. All in all, it is a fairly easy night for the two of us to accumulate seven hours of sleep between us.

Today turns out to be a fairly lax one, and we finish evening rounds at seven. I feel almost as if I were on vacation. Everything is stable at the hospital, easy case for tomorrow, dependable intern on call tonight. Bob and I both decide to go home for the night.

Harriet is glad to see me, my son Ben greets me at the door and with wild excitement explains to me that he has a new baby sister. It feels good to be home with all the family. For the first time in a long while, we spend a leisurely and relaxed evening at home with no calls from the hospital.

The residency progresses, time loses it's meaning and value. I realize I have slowly lost the concept of morning and night. Most people think of going to work in the morning and coming home at night. Even days of the week are lost from the important pages of my mind. I am aware of this time change in my life and wonder if I will ever be able to rearrange my living pattern once residency is completed. The only day that is at all different from any of the rest is Thursday—the day we put in cardiac pacemakers. I look forward to Thursday, mainly because it is a change. I feel I am doing a tremendous service to those patients whose hearts aren't beating at a normal rate, and yet, the procedure is not nearly as time consuming or mentally taxing as operating on the heart.

Today is slack with only one pacemaker, and I decide to give a miniature lecture to the students on our service. We gather in the corner of the diagnostic study room, which is used in putting in the pacemaker. I try to keep my talk informal as I begin to tell about the patients who receive pacemakers.

"Most of the patients have pure, single blockage of the small fibers that carry the impulse through the heart that causes it to beat. This blockage is a significant cause of death in the elderly, estimated to be twelve to thirteen thousand new cases each year in the United States. Thousands of these patients have benefited from the cardiac pacemaker. The idea is simple, and the operation to implant a pacemaker is relatively easy. Normally, there is an area in the atrium of the heart that acts as a transmitter for a small electric impulse to originate. This impulse travels through a system of fibers from the atrium to the ventricle, causing the ventricle to contract each time it is 'shocked,' or stimulated, by the impulse. The ventricle, in turn, reacts by squeezing the blood out of its chamber and thus, causes a 'beat' of the heart. This happens on the average of seventy-two times a minute in a normal, resting individual. Now, that's how it's supposed to work." The students listen intently. There is no note-taking; they will not be given a test on what I am telling them. This is for their own general knowledge of medicine.

"If you take the patient we just operated on, you will see a different picture. The aging process affected his network of conducting fibers and caused them to become scarred and impaired in their duty of 'carrying' the impulse from the atrium to the ventricle. When this happens, the ventricle should theoretically quit beating, since there is nothing there to stimulate it; but like so many other vital systems in the body, there is a back-up system that takes over when the primary one fails. The ventricle begins to beat on its own 'emergency transmitter' at the rate of about forty beats per minute. This rate is fixed and will not increase as the patient exercises or places an increased load on the heart. Such a patient usually has black-out spells due to the fact that not enough blood is being carried to the brain. In the days before artificial pacemakers, the majority of such patients died." I conclude the short lecture on the "blocked heart" and begin to explain the role of the pacemaker.

"The invention of the cardiac pacemaker has drastically changed the outlook of these patients. The pacemaker acts as an artificial transmitting station and consists of two basic parts: the transmitter and the electrodes. The transmitter is a compact unit of stored electrical energy in the form of a battery. An impulse is fired by the transmitter and carried through wires that are connected to the ventrical in some fashion. The wires are electrodes. These electrodes can be carried to the outside of the ventricle, causing a contraction and thus, a beat of the heart. The rate of the pacemaker can be set to a predetermined number per minute.

"As far as actual extension of years in active life, the cardiac pacemaker has probably played a larger role than any other form of surgery related to the heart. There is not nearly the excitement of replacing a heart valve, but the pacemaker implant operation is significant." I finish the short lecture and we start for the x-ray department to view the recent films on our patients. I am actually going to make it home again to eat with my family tonight, unless we find something unusual on rounds.

Two new interns rotate onto the service this month. I dislike the first of the month because they know nothing about our special routine of taking care of post-op heart patients. Not all of them have goals set to include the rough month of our service. As a matter of fact, I am sure some of them have no goals at all. They just want the month to pass. However, by the end of the month most know how to take care of the patients so well, I hate for them to leave. This month, one of the interns who has just started with us has no hope whatsoever of learning how to do *anything* right. John McGill is on every other night, and when he is on Bob and I just have that much more work to do because he can't get the job done. John is on call with us tonight, taking the first opportunity to sit down and light up a cigarette as soon as we finish rounds. Sometimes I feel like taking interns like John aside and explaining to them, that unless they change, they will always be at the bottom of the heap in everything they do. If I could force the goal's book on them, I would, but they wouldn't have the initiative it takes to read it.

"John, get an x-ray on Mrs. Blum in I.C.U. Bob and I have to start the case in the O. R. and will be tied up for awhile. Come down and let us know what the film shows. There hasn't been much blood through the chest tubes, and I want to make sure she isn't pooling it in her chest." I explain as clearly as I know how what I want John to do and why it is important for him to do it.

The usual practice on making rounds is for the intern to write down everything the chief resident wants ordered on each patient and then, following rounds, the intern does the scut work and reports if anything is abnormal. Good interns will take the responsibility of making sure everything on the list is cared for; however, a few will try to get something done on time and if they hit a snag, will let it go. John does not take the responsibility of getting things done. I predict to Bob that the x-ray will not be done when we finish in the O. R. He doesn't understand "Do it now, get it done."

"What did Mrs. Blum's x-ray show?" It is three hours into the evening and Bob and I have just finished our case and walk into the I.C.U. John is standing by the patient I placed a mitral valve in earlier, the patient I asked him to get an x-ray on.

"They haven't gotten the x-ray yet."

"What reason?"

"They have been too busy taking emergencies."

"That . . . is an excuse, not a reason. I bet you don't know the difference between an excuse and a reason. The excuse the x-ray isn't done is that the x-ray girls have been too busy. The reason the x-ray isn't done is because you haven't made it your job to get it done— one way or another." I feel my face flush as my temper rises. The whole problem is immediate action goals. He doesn't understand what action right now means. It is too late to teach him now. The bad part is that he doesn't realize his dilemma. He wouldn't realize what a goal was if it hit him in the face.

If there is one thing I cannot stand. it is not to get something done when given the whole responsibility to do it. Even worse is to blame it on someone else by using the words "they haven't done it." Instead of "I haven't stayed on their backs enough to get it done."

Bob, John, and I walk into the x-ray department to find several patients lying on stretchers waiting to have x-rays taken. I ask why all the backlog and find there are two new technicians on call and they are running at least thirty minutes behind. It is as hopeless to ask one of them to bring a portable machine upstairs to take Mrs. Blum's x-ray as it was to tell John to make sure the film was taken.

"Could I borrow you for just a minute?" I motion one of the girls toward the portable unit. "Write on this paper the settings for a portable film with a patient in a sitting position and at what distance from the patient I should put the machine." If no one else can take the film, I will do it myself, that is, if the technician will go along with my plan.

"You can't take this machine. Besides, we would have to make out the name tags and request forms for the patient, and I am really too busy to do that right now. If you will wait ten minutes, I'll come up and take the film for you."

I turn and direct my question to John. "How long did she say she would be three hours ago?"

"Ten minutes," he replies. At least, he knows how to answer correctly.

Turning back to the technician, I see her pick up a pad and begin writing the instructions to take a portable chest film. "Here are the numbers. Be sure to center it so nothing is hanging over the edges. Destroy the film when you get through because there will not be a name on it and I will get in trouble if they find out an x-ray was taken tonight without proper identification on it." She marches briskly away muttering to herself about her new job and pushy doctors.

I think I am getting the point through to John because when we roll the x-ray unit into the I.C.U. he asks to see the list of instructions for taking the film. He neatly copies them on a wide piece of adhesive tape and affixes the tape inside the cabinet door in I.C.U.: "Instructions On How To Take Chest Film When They Are Too Busy in X-Ray."

There is no blood in Mrs. Blum's chest on x-ray. It has taken me an extra twenty minutes to teach John the meaning of small responsibilities and how to handle immediate action goals. Whether it will ever be profitable to him in the future, I don't know. In John's case, I doubt it. Trying to teach an individual who has no goals is like trying to cut with a knife that has no blade. There will always be people like John who will never need a *Goal's Rule Book*. These people are satisfied with what they have. They set no goals, will rarely do what they are told to do, never do more than is expected of them—only the amount of work they are paid to do and feel cheated if they don't get paid for any extra work they perform. John is one of these people. But because there are so many Johns in the world, *everyone* who takes it upon himself to work on goals will be successful. I'll bet at least ninety percent of people are just like John, with no known goals in life. If this is true, it means only ten percent are really striving to get ahead. Simple deduction is all I need to conclude that anyone who decides to set goals and jump into this ten percent group will become successful according to his goals. Even if he falls to the bottom of the ten percent pile, he will still be ahead of ninety percent of everyone else.

I pull out my well-worn *Goal's Rule Book*, from my pocket and write on the last page: The Ninety Percent Rule: No goals, no competition. Remember the Johns in life. Set goals and join the top ten percent.

The time for me to remain chief resident is drawing to a close. In only a few more months, I will no longer be a resident. Much has transpired since that first day in medical school sitting at a desk, thinking about a structure to develop in order to get through medical school and become a surgeon. One thing I do realize is that the resultant framework of goals I developed has made a big change in my life. Almost every action I make is made from habit. I have been able to change my life; to control my life by making habits. The rules have slowly changed into habits. Repetition of the rules has led to automatic habits. No longer do I have to refer back to my rules. They have become so imprinted in my mind that I react automatically. That is the missing link that joins it all together. Set the major goal, make your rules, persist in them until they become habit.

I awaken to the fact I need to get on down to the pediatric ward to see Greg Wilson, our next open-heart case. Greg is five years old and is being admitted for a work-up of congenital aortic stenosis, tightness of one of the heart valves since birth, and the work-up entails cardiac catheterization and injecting some dye into the heart in an attempt to visualize just how tight the valve is.

He is too young to have the valve excised and an artificial one put in place; we will have to try to open his congenitally small valve and make it function a few more years until his heart grows large enough to accept an artificial valve.

Greg sits on the floor playing with some toys when I walk in to examine him. This is an exceptionally difficult case for me to work on because I know Greg's father and mother from our church. Greg and my son are in the same Sunday school class. This will be the first time I will have ever operated on anyone I have personally known. We are not close friends, but I know the family, have empathy for what they are about to go through. I question Greg's mother about his symptoms.

"He hasn't really been very sick," she tells me. "He does get short of breath if he plays hard, but the heart medicine he takes pretty well keeps him out of trouble."

Greg glances up at me and smiles. At his age, he can enjoy the blessed innocence concerning worry of everyday happenings; to him life and death operations are incomprehensible. Mr. Wilson and I have talked about Greg's upcoming operation on several occasions; how it will not be a very long procedure, how Greg will have to be placed on the heart-lung pump only long enough to open the aortic valve—not much of an operation at all, relative to other heart surgery. It all sounds very simple and straightforward to discuss the case, but we both are aware that any time the heart is operated on, numerous events can occur that potentially could prove fatal. The chances of this happening are slim, but ever-present.

"Greg, slip your shirt off and let me listen to your heart." He is a well-mannered boy who immediately pulls his shirt off over his head and comes over to where I can examine him. I place my hand on his sternum and feel a fine vibration with each beat of his heart, indicating a turbulence of blood flow as it passes through the valve. Placing my stethoscope over the region of the aortic valve, I hear the harsh sound of blood being forcefully ejected through an opening in a valve which should be large enough to accept the end of the index finger. As I listen, I picture the small, contracted hole, only a fraction as large as it should be. I hope this will be a case in which the noise the blood makes as it crosses the constricted valve is relatively louder than the severity of the tightness of the valve.

Greg undergoes cardiac catheterization and the results are disheartening. The opening in the valve is minute compared to what it should be. He goes home to await his surgery which is planned for June.

He is allowed to visit his grandparents the weekend before coming back into the hospital and enjoys an early birthday party with them. Little Greg and his teddy bear are equally unaware of all that is taking place. It is senseless to try to explain the danger he is about to face; how much pain he will have after the operation; the tubes coming out of his chest; the tubes in the veins of his neck and arms; the wires and gadgets connected to his body to record his heart beat, the tube in his bladder to measure the hourly output of urine; or the doctors and nurses constantly around him checking for any post-operative abnormalities. To tell Greg all this will only scare him, although we do show him the intensive care unit he will be placed in after leaving the recovery room. Perhaps this will alleviate some of the fear he will be required to face all alone.

"The same age as my son." I cannot get this off my mind. Why should a boy this young have to suffer anything so painful and stressful as a heart operation? I have to force myself not to get involved with the unanswerable questions concerning this case. I am a surgeon, not a philosopher; the more time I spend philosophizing, the less time I have to prepare for the operation.

We start the case at seven A.M. and everything goes well. We place a tube into the femoral artery in the leg and another into the veins going into the heart, connect them to the heart-lung machine in order to make a closed circuit between Greg and the machine.

"Let's go on," the familiar words instruct the technician to start the pump to begin the blood flowing out of the right atrium and into the heart-lung machine in order for oxygenation to be accomplished. The pump is started and begins to "push" the blood back into the body via the femoral artery. A clamp is placed across the aorta near the malformed valve to keep blood from flooding the operative field once the aorta is opened. An incision is made in the aorta and the valve inspected.

"Look at that valve!" Dr. Bell shakes his head in disbelief. The valve area has no resemblance to an aortic valve, but looks like a clump of smooth, shining tissue resembling "Silly Putty." It has no shape or form. Usually there are three cusps, or cups, making up the aortic valve, and all that needs to be done is to cut between each cup to increase the diameter of the opening. "I don't know if we are going to be able to do much to this valve. It has the look of one you would expect to see at an autopsy in an infant who died from aortic stenosis. That's no valve. It's just embryonic tissues clumped together. I don't see how he has lived this long." Dr. Bell is amazed that the heart could have used this valve for any purposeful effect.

We examine the valve closer and, since there are no identifiable cusps, decide to make a two-leafed valve out of it by placing two small incisions opposite each other. We are walking a tightrope with this boy's life and everything has to go one hundred percent correctly or we will surely lose him.

We make the incisions in the valve.

Close the aorta.

Release the clamp on the aorta.

Begin to slow the pump in order to let the heart take over and pump more of the blood on its own.

"Let's go off." The pump is stopped and Greg's heart takes over perfectly. "Pump time" has been nine minutes—not bad, considering the fact we had to alter the routine of incising the valve and decide exactly where and how to incise.

Dr. Bell drops out of the case since everything is stable and goes to explain to the parents what we found and what has been done. A future operation will be needed because the valve will have to be replaced as soon as the heart grows large enough to accept an artificial valve. It isn't good news, but at least we have done enough to keep his heart going until that time comes for another operation.

We take Greg to the recovery room and begin the all important post-operative monitoring. The first thirty minutes go well, but all of a sudden the cardiac monitor shows something irregular, more irregular—ventricular fibrillation. The heart only quivers and loses all effectiveness in beating. I immediately begin external massage as Dr. Bell gives orders to get the pump ready immediately. I crawl up on his bed and continue the massage as we roll him back to the O.R. The incision is quickly reopened and we work frantically to place him back on the pump. We operate for two hours, knowing all the time fate is against us. With a valve like this one in his heart, and the ventricle fibrillating, the chance of pulling him through is almost nil. A lump comes to my throat as we repeatedly fail to get him off the pump. I cannot talk. My eyes are watery as I stare at the dying heart. I feel helpless. We are doing everything we know to do, but still we can not make Greg's heart beat again. I desperately try to think of something to do that may pull him through. I know Dr. Bell is rerunning every conceivable thought through his mind that may produce an answer as how to get the heart to work again.

"God, you can't let this happen. Why don't You do something? Can't You understand we're losing him. We're losing Greg!" I half pray and half think to myself. I become deaf to all the talking around me. Dr. Bell gives further instructions and we follow through with them, but nothing registers in my mind. We have lost him. We try to get him off the pump a few more times, but each time his heart is not strong enough to take over.

Why are we operating so long this time? Dr. Bell knows, and I know, that our chances of getting him back, sank to less than one percent after the first thirty minutes lapsed and his heart continued deteriorating. By all logic, we both are convinced that all hope is gone; yet I can visualize Greg's heart coming back on its own and beating without the aid of the pump, can visualize Greg's parents being told that everything is all right, that Greg is going to make it. Still, these thoughts can only be fantasy, but for us to give up is to end the life of a child. Only when that one percent of hope is exhausted, will Dr. Bell give the order. Only then will we have paid our debt to death in our minds.

"Turn the pump off." It is all over. We have failed to get the heart going again. Dr. Bell says he will go speak to the family. I start closing the chest. This time there is no pulsating heart pounding under the incision; no need to worry about making sure all vessels are tied off to control bleeding. Nothing matters now. Greg is no longer with us. His body is still here, but Greg isn't. How do you explain death to a mother and father when you don't understand it yourself.

A strange quietness falls over the room with no one saying a word. The anesthesiologist is busy gathering his equipment. He isn't needed for the closure of the wound this time. A scrub nurse stays and passes suture as I need it, but no words are exchanged. A plastic bag is brought in for the body. I finish closing the skin, remove my gloves and head for the on-call room to be alone.

I sit on the left side of the bed and stare at a blank wall. The only word I can think of is: "Why." For one hour I sit with an occasional tear running down my face. High school, yes, that was the last time I cried, and I can't even remember the reason now. It was so insignificant I can't even remember why. But this is so different. Now I play the game of life and death with humans. I lay back on the bed and close my eyes. All I can see is that valve. "Embryonic valve," I keep thinking. "Never saw anyone live this long with a valve like that." Dr. Bell had said. I remember his saying just that. I open my eyes. Maybe Greg should have died as an infant, or even before. Maybe Greg's parents had a few years of happiness with him when by all facts and figures he should have died sooner. I try to reason, but cannot. All I know is that Greg Wilson was playing with some early birthday toys yesterday and now, those toys will never again be played with by him.

I hear my name being paged for Dr. Bell's office. I elect to go on down to talk with him in person rather than over the phone.

He is sitting at his desk as I enter. He straightens a few mis-aligned papers on his desk and pushes back in his chair in preparation for speaking. He holds his chin between his thumb and fore-finger and sights in on the corner of his desk as I've seen him do so often before when he is getting ready to talk of a serious matter.

"There is one thing you cannot do in surgery—if you have done the best you can—and that is to blame yourself for the death of a patient. You did your best; I did my best. Greg's valve was so borderline, it couldn't take the added strain of an operation, especially one which didn't really help the dynamics of the heart all that much." Dr. Bell realizes the mental beating I have taken since the operation. He has been there before and is much the wiser for it.

I still cannot speak, only listen. He continues, "You have rounds to make, x-rays to see, patients to care for, and interns to give instructions to. It is best you get back to work. We will get together in the morning and rehash the case to see if there was something we could have done differently."

I nod in the affirmative and leave his office. I am sick of going over deaths to see what could have been done differently. I am tired of M&M conferences. I don't want to discuss deaths and complications. I don't want to make rounds with the residents and interns. I don't want to look at x-rays. I don't want to follow any of the crazy rules I have set up for myself concerning pushing on, going the extra mile, getting it done. Right now, all is futile. The whole rotten structure of goals and residency and medicine stinks. I am mentally beat. I am going home.

The experience of previous years tells me I cannot simply leave without making sure the service is in order, so I tell Bob to take charge of rounds, that I will return later tonight to see the patients by myself, to call me at home if any troubles come up.

I give my son an extra hug and kiss when I make it home. He doesn't understand why I hold him so long. I can't explain the action to him or the reason I do not talk with him. Harriet knows which case I had scheduled for today and senses it didn't go well.

"Did something go wrong with the operation?"

"Wrong is not the word for it. Greg didn't make it." I sit down and pretend I am looking at the newspaper. Harriet sits beside me and says nothing. Finally she says, "I'm sorry." She squeezes my hand before going into the bedroom to check on Patricia.

She is sorry, but there is no way for her to really understand the feeling. Ben is busy playing with his toy cars. There is no way he can have any understanding of what has taken place. Greg Wilson's parents have lost their son. They are grieved and hurt. But even they cannot understand my feelings now. A life is entrusted into your hands and in a few short hours, that life is no longer. How can a surgeon learn to cope with this?

"Come on and eat. You will feel better when you get some food in your stomach." Harriet knows at least one way to make me feel better. I go to the table with no appetite, but I eat.

I return to the hospital for some quick rounds and then crawl into bed for some much needed sleep. Even Patricia's crying does not wake me.

I awake in the morning and find I do not want to return to work. Thinking about the hospital puts a bad taste in my mouth, but I automatically pull out the bad apple rule from the book, throw out that bad apple thought, and replace it with the thought of reality. I am almost through residency and that is a reward worth going back to the hospital for. I have to pull all my habits back together, throw out the bad thoughts of yesterday, feed in the good thoughts of tommorow. The bad apple rule involves only one thing: *attitude.* How I handle this situation and all other "bad apple" situations depends one hundred percent on attitude, and attitude is the one thing over which I have one hundred percent control.

I have been rewarded with a full night's sleep because there was no open-heart case to stay up with, an ironic prize for the death of a patient. The night's rest brings clearer thinking, however, about the life and death aspect of surgery. I make as the immediate action goal of today to once again start following the rules I have set down for myself as a resident. Last night was the only time during my entire training that I have not adhered to the rules I have set up. I concede to that one defeat, but I am back in the game this morning to win by the rules.

I enter the last month of residency with all the feeling of competency I had following my year as an intern. It is truly remarkable that a medical student can start in a training period of surgery as soon as he completes medical school and come out, a few years later, a surgeon. I accept the fact that it takes some intelligence to be accepted to medical school, but after that it is almost directly related to how much work you put into it that determines where you come out in the field of medicine. This idea is even more true in the field of surgery. So much of my training has been pure hard work and long hours. The academic portion is there to be learned and all it takes is time to learn it. At this stage of the game, I look back to decide if I have managed my time successfully. The few weeks that remain will be insignificant relative to all the hours already spent learning to become a surgeon. I turn all the cases over to Bob the last two weeks with the exception of one case I have wanted to perform since the first day I decided to take the cardio-thoracic residency: a triple valve operation.

Dr. Bell is going to give me the opportunity to do what I have seen and read about but never thought I would ever actually perform. I am scheduled to remove three of the four valves in Mrs. Maude Vaughn's heart and replace them with three artificial ones. Our patient has rheumatic disease in these valves and all three need replacing with prostheses. Dr. Bell has me scheduled as the first surgeon, and I know the only way I will come out with a live patient following an operation of this magnitude, is to perform it without a technical mistake.

I stand at the scrub sink this morning thinking of what has brought me to this point in my career. I am almost through my surgical training, have matured surgically and mentally, have learned, have formed habits, good and bad. I think of one habit that has happened by chance more than planning. I remember back to the day I performed my first hernia operation at the V. A. hospital as a junior medical student and cannot recall whether I was afraid of not doing a good job or whether I wanted to help. But while scrubbing my hands, I said a jumbled prayer simply asking that I do my best on that case. I have never performed an operation since, when I have not repeated that prayer. Today is no different. The only significance lies in the fact that I started with a simple hernia operation, and today I am to replace three valves inside a heart.

I begin the operation by removing the heavily calcified aortic valve and sewing the artificial valve in place. Next comes the mitral valve which goes as planned. I am making good time and have a chance to get the patient off the pump without prolonged bypass time if I can get the tricuspid valve cut out and replaced without undue delay. The longer the patient is on the pump, the greater chance there is for difficulty in getting her heart to beat on its own. So far, so good.

All is quiet in the room. The scrub nurse hasn't said two words since we started. I haven't had to lift my eyes from the operative field; the nurse has everything ready as I need it. I feel the quietness. Everything goes better without all the gab that usually is present in the operating room. If I had my way, the mask covering our faces would mute words coming out of the mouth in addition to cutting down on the number of bacteria extruded.

I open the right atrium and find a large, dilated chamber which was made so by back leakage of blood through the incompetent valve. Such a large atrium makes it easy to work in, but it also means the atrium has been greatly overworked in order to have attained such a large size.

The tricuspid valve is excised and the new one put in place. Mrs. Vaughn comes off the bypass without difficulty and it looks as if she is going to do nicely on her own.

"Excellent!" Dr. Bell uses one word of praise following the case.

Excellent. What I have gone through for that one word to be muttered to me one time. Initially, I am flattered, but as I have time to think of the word, I begin to realize that it is not me he is talking to. Not the individual "self." He is talking to practice and experience—two entities that anyone can obtain with enough stamina to stick to it. With this simple understanding, my ego deflates as rapidly as it had inflated. The compliment from Dr. Bell drops from a ten rating down to a one. I have arrived as a surgeon. I no longer need compliments from my colleagues in order to do a good job. The patient is sick; I operate on him and that is that. There is no need for

— 211 —

anyone to be in the grandstand cheering, or observing, or interested in what I am doing; it is down to a surgical relationship between me and the patient. In the past ten minutes I have come to realize what a real surgeon is all about. It has nothing to do with competition between interns and residents, it doesn't matter what your assistant thinks about the way you handle a knife and a pair of scissors; it is insignificant for the head of the service to pay you a compliment. The truth lies only in how well the patient does as a direct result of the way I perform an operation.

This realization is almost anticlimatic. A year earlier, if Dr. Bell or Dr. Eler had paid me such a compliment, I could have hardly waited to tell Bob First about it, or tell Harriet immediately after getting home. Now, it only registers in my mind, to remain untold.

Two days pass. Mrs. Vaughn is doing well with no complications.

I sit at the side of her bed in I.C.U. to have an informal chat about how she is doing. I ask her if she can tolerate a few more days with all the wires and tubes coming out of her.

"They don't bother me," she replies. "What *is* getting to me, is the clicking of the valves in my heart. You didn't tell me I would be able to hear them click. It's going to drive me crazy. Everytime I wake up, all I can hear are those valves clicking."

"Don't worry about the clicking; you'll get used to that. The time to start worrying is when you *don't* hear the clicking." I reassure her.

I relate the incident to Dr. Bell later in the day, and he informs me there have been suicides attributed to the clicking sound of the artificial valves—sort of like a water faucet dripping as you are trying to get some sleep. The only problem is the patient can't get up and turn it off.

The third night post-operatively, "500, I.C.U.," "500, I.C.U." comes over the intercom. Mrs. Vaughn. I know it's her. There has been too much done for her to come through the operation without a single complication.

I run up the six flights of stairs to the I.C.U. to see a resusitation already in progress on Mrs. Vaughn.

"What happened?" The intern is giving external massage and the general surgery resident who was in the I.C.U. at the time is just finishing placing an endotracheal tube into her trachea.

"Her pulse rate went to zero. I heard the monitor buzz and looked over and didn't see a thing on the scope," the nurse explains as she hangs an Isuprel drip in the I.V. to stimulate the heart to beat more rapidly.

"Let's see what she has on the monitor." I motion for the intern to stop the external massage. It shows a regular rhythm and I place my hand on her groin to feel the pulse. Strong and full. Her heart is back on its own and beating normally. Mrs. Vaughn opens her eyes and looks at me without moving from her position on the cardiac arrest board under her back.

"You're O.K. Your heart is beating normally. You are going to be all right. I'll take that tube out of your windpipe in a little while. Your heart stopped beating for a minute but it looks good now." I reassure her that everything is all right, but I wonder myself exactly what happened. Why did her heart stop beating, and why is it beating normally now? Did the nurse actually check to see if the heart had quit or did she just glance at the monitor and think the heart had stopped? I've had numerous cardiac arrests after open-heart surgery, but never had one that has gone like this one. There was not five minutes work done and now the heart is beating normally as ever. The cardiogram looks the same as this time yesterday. After an hour of observation on the monitor, I see what is happening. Her heart slows to a rate of forty, I give Isuprel and the rate picks back up to eighty. It now becomes obvious what is happening. The conduction fibers in the heart that carry the beating impulse from the atrium to the ventricle are not working. She is having heart block, just like the elderly patients who require pacemakers. However, the cause for this blockage is different. The blockage has to be surgically related to sewing in the last valve.

The solution to the problem is to put a cardiac pacemaker in to control her rate. I explain the situation to Mrs. Vaughn and return her to the operating room and put a pacemaker on her heart. She does well following this. Upon discharging her from the hospital I have a feeling of accomplishment that can come only after the years of surgical training which has led me to this point in life.

I complete my last week of residency in a state of complete satisfaction with my life, with my work, and with my future. I come to the hospital the last day of work to say goodbyes more than anything else. I have made friends who I will never forget. Many incidents and many patients will remain in my memory, needing only a small reminder to bring them forth. There is no way to offer the thanks deserved by Dr. Bell and Dr. Eler, but I make an effort to tell them what their teaching and training has meant to me. There is joking and kidding with the other residents and interns, and we talk quickly of how each will remember the other. As at all times like this, we only mention the good, the fun parts, the successful operations we performed together. We exchange many "remember the time" incidents we have lived through over the past several years. And, sticking to the ritual, we promise to get together again soon and keep in touch.

Before leaving the hospital for the last time, I go by the "office" where Bob and I spent so much time to pick up my belongings. I leave my old razor, shaving cream, shampoo, and toothpaste. I am sure they will all be used by someone within a week.

I sit down on the edge of the bed and smile as I glance at the framed Murphy's Laws. Talk about negative thinking! I scoot back on the bed and prop my back against the wall. I take a small worn notebook from my right hand coat pocket and thumb through it. The *Goal's Rule Book* has proven successful. It has stood the test of time through medical school, internship, and surgical residency. There is no doubt in my mind that whatever major goal I decide to set, I can reach. Just as I understood anatomy in medical school, I understand goal anatomy with one exception. The reason I know I can personally achieve any major goal I set is because of some power within my mind that will never let me set an unattainable major goal. What this power is, I do not know, but I do know if I can think of it, I can do it. Furthermore, it is a simple matter to reach a major goal by staying within the framework of the *Goal's Rule Book*. The major goal depends upon the intermediate goals, and the intermediate goals depend upon immediate action goals, and the simple fact that the immediate action goals mean action RIGHT NOW. The price to pay for reaching any major goal is the cost of the immediate action goals. This can be very costly. It can cost time from family, time from leisure activity, time from sleep; but the solution is simple. If willing to pay that cost absolutely, any goal that your mind will let you set can be reached successfully.

I make one last entry, something I saw on a poster one time. "Happy is the man who sets a goal and is willing to pay the price to reach it." I do feel happy. I have paid the price. The race is over. I am ready for the reward that Harriet and I have talked about so much—free time.

I leave the hospital shortly after noon. I walk out the front door alone and glance around. There should be a band playing. It seems there really ought to be someone standing on the front lawn waving flags. There should be crowds cheering. I have just finished years of study which required dedication, and even now, I don't see how I did it. I am so full of happiness I feel I may explode. I want to tell everyone. I have a smile on my face that won't change to anything else. I have just conquered the biggest goal I could possibly set in my life.

But I walk on alone, and no one seems to notice. Two young boys are playing out by the spraying fountain in front of the hospital. Patients continue to come up the walk and pass me without fanfare. This is real. This is life. No one here can experience my joy. They have not experienced my life up to this moment and can have no empathy with me now.

"Sir, can you tell me where the interns are supposed to meet this morning?" A one-day-old intern stops me and brings my mind back to reality.

"You don't know?" I ask almost in disbelief. "Go to Dr. Eler's office and ask the secretary. She will get you straightened out."

I stand a moment and watch him walk away. He has a long road ahead of him. Maybe I should have given him my *Goal's Rule Book*.

Part VI

THE FINALE

ONCE MY SURGICAL TRAINING is completed, I enter the Air Force for a two-year stint. There is so much free time, actually some time to spend with the family, time to do some things I have wanted to do. I recall all of those nights in training where I would lie in bed and, just before drifting off to sleep, think of being outside and doing things my mind made me believe I could do. I take up flying, become more active in mountain climbing, even start sky-diving. I feel like a bird out of a cage. The one sport that will require all of the goal structure I have developed in surgical training is one I desire to learn the most: kayaking. Before even seeing a real kayak, I set running the Colorado River through the Grand Canyon as a MAJOR GOAL. I know this is the ultimate in kayak-running, comprising some of the most challenging rapids in the world that only the apex of the pyramid system of kayakers are ever able to run. For an INTERMEDIATE GOAL I pick the Green River, which runs through Dinosaur National Monument in Utah. It is a river with several big holes and waves that will require some expertise, but not on a scale as large as the Grand Canyon. Now for the hard part—IMMEDIATE ACTION GOAL, the "right now" part: build a kayak, get in a pool and learn to roll back up after turning over, get in some moving water, find some small rapids to learn in, throw myself into some holes in the river and see what happens; start learning, doing, aiming for the MAJOR GOAL—the Grand.

I hold onto the goal structure that proved so valuable in getting through surgical training and that continues to ring true in my life outside surgery. I build a kayak, go to a pool and learn to roll, get in some rapids and learn how a river speaks softly and loud, tiptoes along and runs. I make it down the Green River in Dinosaur and finally spend two weeks in the Grand Canyon getting eaten alive by giant holes. But I make it and another MAJOR GOAL is accomplished.

Life is so exciting, so full, so rewarding . . . yet, something is missing. The pastor of the church Harriet and I have joined talks of a full and meaningful life. I begin to ask myself questions about how wonderful my life is under the present goal system. I begin to discuss this "full and meaningful" situation with my kayaking buddies. One day I am on the river with a surgeon friend who had climbed into the goal system of running the Grand Canyon with me. We begin to discuss the topic of "goals" and basic Christianity.

"Larry, we set goals to make it through the Grand Canyon and now continue to reap enjoyment kayaking river after river. You mentioned some time ago that you were a Christian. I call myself a Christian. Yet, we get together on the river and set goals in medicine; we talk about goals in investments and goals for our children; but we have never talked about setting any goals concerning what we ought to be doing for Christ." I speak during one of our frequent stops to scout an upcoming rapid. Larry stops, unsnaps his wet-suit top, pulls his helmet off, and sits down on a clump of grass on the riverbank. We have never discussed religion, nor politics, to any depth. I am not sure how he is going to handle such a question—a shrug of shoulders, a smile, or a let's-change-the-subject attitude.

"I know what you are saying," he replies. "Jesus said to 'feed my sheep' and all I am doing is feeding myself. Tell you what. Let's both start right now asking God what we ought to be doing for Him." Larry talks of what has been on his mind for some time, of what has been unspoken because there was no one to talk to about it.

I start to dissect the flaws and pitfalls of the goal system scheme I so carefully put together in surgical training, pointing out to Larry, "You know the *Goal's Rule Book* I told you about that I put together during training? Well, that same plan of setting a MAJOR GOAL, INTERMEDIATE GOAL, AND IMMEDIATE ACTION GOAL could be used by someone who has decided to rob a bank. He could take the outline I have set up and become the best, most successful, most accomplished, most wealthy bank robber around. Something is missing. The same plan shouldn't be able to work for us and for a bank robber. The missing ingredient must be what my pastor keeps talking about—Christ living through us, our actions, our plans, our goals."

As months pass, I recall very little about the holes, the rapids, the excitement on the river that day with Larry. But a thought keeps coming back to me about our discussion. What is the difference between me and that bank robber I talked about? I don't know the difference but I know the similarity. His goal structure and mind are both centered on "self." Somehow "self" has to be put aside in my life and replaced by Christ, the one who will set the goals and center my actions. This reasoning makes me review the basic goal structure I have set down for myself and see where the flaw leading to success may be.

Step one: Visualize having accomplished the set goal. I remember seeing myself as a surgeon years before I ever became one.

Step two: Write down the goal and what I have to do to reach it. I can remember writing down intermediate and immediate action goals time and time again in order to ingrain them into my mind. Writing it down is seen as an essential part of goal-setting.

Step three: Commit myself to that goal. Pay whatever price I have to pay but never turn back. Burn every bridge behind me. Decide the goal can be accomplished and replace any negative thought about that goal with a positive one. Total commitment is essential.

Step four: Remind myself of the goal daily. Write the goal down on an index card and carry it in my billfold. Tape it to my shaving mirror. Place it on my night stand so I can read it before going to bed. I remember the first year Harriet and I were married. I had sutures tied to the refrigerator handle, to the door handle, to the back of chairs. Each suture was a visual reminder to me of my goal of becoming a surgeon.

Step five: Allow for roadblocks. There is no set goal that will ever be reached without a multitude of stumbling blocks in the road. Expect them. Prepare for them with persistence of mind. Keep an eye on the goal and begin to work around the obstacle. Persist, persist, persist. In internship, when I sat alone in the on-call room and thought about applying for another surgical residency program, one that was easier, I faced a boulder in the road. I had two choices: turn back from the difficult surgery program and seek an easier one; or face the boulder, persist until I could see my mind clearly enough to realize I had what it took to reach the goal of remaining in Dr. Eller's residency. Accept the fact of boulders in the path. Push them out of the way.

Step six: The major goal is accomplished only one stitch at a time. The goal seems so big, so unattainable, so far away that it appears impossible for me to reach. The bricklayer of a skyscraper places one brick at a time. When I did my first hernia operation, I thought it was the biggest procedure in the world. Yet, when I saw a chief resident taking out part of a man's aorta I realized there was no way in the world I could do that operation at the time. It seemed so far in the future to me. How would I ever be able to do such an operation? One stitch at a time. Visualize the goal and work on it one stitch at a time.

This has been the anatomy of my goal structure in the past. It should lead to success. Is success really just the process of setting a goal, working toward it, and finally accomplishing it? Until now, I think that has been the way I have looked at success. But there is one problem. What about the successful businessman who has everything a person can ask for and yet does not have inner peace? His inner world is falling apart. What about the individual who forfeits his family time, free time, time alone with his wife—all for success in his business? When it is all over and this man has lost his family and stepped on his friends, but has accomplished his goals in his business endeavors, is he successful? There lies the difference. There lies the flaw in my goal structure for success. He is not successful, he has only accomplished his goals. What I have set up is a goal structure for making accomplishments. You can take the goal structure and accomplish anything you set as a goal. That will work. I am sure of it. All of this time I have been working toward accomplishing goals rather than becoming a success. The difference has to be centered around God's direction on my goals. Accomplishments versus success —there is a difference.

The months extend into years and I start down a long road of searching, asking questions, seeking, reading. I finish my Air Force commitment and enter the private practice of surgery with my brother. After some time passes I hear of a Billy Graham crusade coming to a nearby town. My brother and I decide to attend and there meet a man who is on the Billy Graham team. He begins telling us he has a son, a surgeon in India, who needs help from surgeons willing to leave their practice for four to six weeks at a time and operate at the mission hospital where he works.

The new structure of goals begin to unfold slowly. I come across a scripture that can be used as the MAJOR GOAL at all times: Love the Lord your God with all your heart, with all your soul, with all your mind—Matthew 22:37.

It soon becomes settled. My brother and I will go to India and serve as surgeons for four to six weeks.

Once there, it is evident that many more surgeons than my brother and myself are needed. Also, numerous mission hospitals are in dire need of surgeons to relieve the full-time doctor who needs a month off for rest or simply just to ease his caseload for a while. My brother and I decide for once in our lives to let God call the shots, to let Him plan what we should do. We begin a small organization to try to encourage other surgeons to tithe their time and talents in the mission field and relieve full-time doctors.

Billy Graham's son, Franklin, hears of our work and accepts the challenge of finding these surgeons who will work with us. One goal leads to another. Now, however, there is something vastly different. There is the most powerful peace describable in my life; no anxious moments, no scheming to be done. The goals become different; a new perspective emerges. I still jump at a challenge like a dog to a rabbit, still set goals and still have dreams. But the underlying theme changes. It is a difficult change for me.

"How many surgeons a year do you think you can get to go to the mission field for short-term help?" Franklin asks my brother and me as we discuss the future of the newly formed organization called World Medical Missions.

"If we could get five or ten a year, we would be doing well," I respond.

"What would be wrong with a goal of fifty?" Franklin fires back. "If you really turn this over to the Lord, and let Him work through you, there is no telling how He will utilize all of us."

So, that's how it is. MAJOR GOAL, INTERMEDIATE GOAL, IMMEDIATE GOAL, right now or later; it matters little if they are misguided goals. All goals must become redirected goals, must be brought into the proper perspective, must become new creatures, new goals.

The goal structure remains the same; dreams are turned into goals and goals into reality. But I find an even larger factor that can change our lives lies in the biggest Goal Book of all: the Bible. Consider II Corinthians 5:17: Therefore, if anyone is in Christ, he is a new creature; the old has gone, the new has come!

Dreams, goals, reality; the new can come.